BECOME A
BETTER YOU

BECOME A BETTER YOU

BETTER YOU

STOP DIETING, START LIVING

BYRON MORRISON

This book is a general educational health-related information product and is intended for healthy adults, aged 18 and over.
This book is solely for information and educational purposes and is not medical advice. Please consult a medical or health professional before you begin any exercise, nutrition, or supplementation program, or if you have questions about your health.

There may be risks associated with participating in activities or using products mentioned in this book for people in poor health or with pre-existing physical or mental health conditions.

Because these risks exist, you will not use such products or participate in such activities if you are in poor health or have a pre-existing mental or physical health condition. If you choose to participate in these activities, you do so of your own free will and accord knowingly and voluntarily, assuming all risks associated with such activities.

Specific results mentioned in this book should be considered extraordinary and there are no "typical" results. As individuals differ, then results will differ.

Cover designed by: Julia Protesaru

Typesetting by: Byron Morrison

Edited by: Julia Protesaru

Published by: Tailored Lifestyles

Visit the author's website: www.tailoredlifestyles.co.uk

ISBN: 978-1-5272-0439-3

First Edition: November 2016

Dedication

This book is dedicated to my parents, who without none of this would have been possible.

Thank you for your ongoing endless support and belief, as I wouldn't be where I am today or the person I am without you.

And to Jules, for all the long hours, late nights and endless patience in helping make this a reality.

Contents

About the author

Hi, my name is Byron Morrison, thanks for picking up a copy of my book, Become a Better You.

Before we begin, I'd like to just tell you a little about myself, how I came to write this book, my reasons for doing so and what we will be covering. Hopefully this will give you a better understanding of who I am, along with my goals and mission as both an author and a lifestyle coach, in turn helping you make up your own mind as to whether or not you should listen to me.

So what's my story?

I know that change is hard, in fact, I know exactly how daunting and overwhelming it can be. Just like most people I used to struggle with the entire concept of what a healthier lifestyle is all about and why it's so important. I paid no attention to what I did or ate, living a largely sedentary life comprising of little to no physical activity and a diet filled with highly refined and processed foods. Spending my days mostly indoors, glued to the latest shows and video games, completely unaware and oblivious to the long-term damage I was causing, and it showed, on a mental, physical and emotional level. I was nearly 50 pounds heavier, and had huge problems with everything from self-confidence to managing stress and my relationships with food. Even my mindset was affected, skewing the way I dealt with the ups and downs of everyday life, and having a tremendous impact on my overall outlook. The truth is I never realised how bad I felt until I finally started to feel better, and that's the unfortunate reality so many people are living in every day.

It wasn't until I nearly lost my dad to cancer and saw the pain and suffering he went through during the treatment (including 25 days in ICU, having most of his bowel surgically removed, being placed on life support and kept alive through the use breathing machines on two separate occasions, as well has having a tracheostomy) that it dawned on me how much of an influence his lifestyle choices had on causing the disease. From a diet high in sugar and processed foods, to being a pack-a-day smoker who did no exercise, all combined with having an overwhelmingly stressful career, working 14-hour days, with a minimal amount of sleep, it's no surprise it took a toll on his health.

That was the point I decided I needed to change, so I spent the next few years researching everything I could about health, fitness, nutrition and general wellbeing. I studied everything from the benefits of fuelling our body with what it actually requires, to how diseases could be cured, treated or even prevented through proper nutrition, the psychological factors influencing the daily decisions we make, the importance of exercise and the negative effects our lifestyle choices and habits have on our health. I spent hours every day reading books, scientific studies, watching documentaries, studying testimonials and gaining qualifications to back it all up.

Through this learning process I realised the general population's knowledge and understanding of health and nutrition is minimal at best, and it could even be argued that in many cases what people do know is so wildly misguided, that it's actually detrimental to their health. After all, I was a prime example of the average member of society, only really knowing we should be aiming to be more active and eat our fruits and vegetables. I was clueless about how processed, refined and sugar-filled the products we eat actually are, let alone how much of a direct impact they have on our overall health. I also had no idea how to put together a balanced diet, which when you think about it, is something that really should be a basic life skill, and I never even considered the impact my mindset and ever growing stress levels were having on my wellbeing.

The problem is there's so much bad information out there, which is why my goal is to pass on the knowledge that I have learned, to help people make more informed decisions on how to improve their lives and their families. A healthy lifestyle really is a choice that is not only achievable, but also sustainable, and it is my hope that I can help others avoid going through what happened to my dad.

I know embarking on this journey is a daunting prospect, but I honestly believe that if I can do it, then so can you. I am living proof it can be done, which is why I have designed this process around the guidance, information and support I wish had back when I was struggling to get started .

With that being said, whether you read my book, are part my coaching services, or simply someone who stumbled onto my website, I'm happy to help in any way that I can. That's why I dedicate a few hours each day to answering questions on a range of topics from health to nutrition, dieting, fitness, and general wellbeing. All I ask in return is if you like the content I'm creating, then please share it with your family and friends. The only way we are going to create substantial change on a national level is to inform and help educate as many people as possible, even if that means starting with one person at a time.

That's why I offer a free, no obligation 'start your weight loss journey' break through session over Skype, where we can discuss the issues you are facing and I can help you put together a plan on how to get started.

You can book your session now at:
www.tailoredlifestyles.co.uk/breakthrough

Or you can contact me directly at:
byron@tailoredlifestyles.co.uk

Alternatively, you can use the community discussed later in this book, or follow me on any of the social media platforms listed below:
http://www.facebook.com/tailoredlifestyles
https://uk.linkedin.com/in/byronmorrisontl
https://www.instagram.com/tailoredlifestyles

I hope you enjoy this book for what I hope it will be: an eye-opening, educational journey, that will finally give you the knowledge, inspiration and guidance to have the health, prosperity and lifestyle you have always wanted.

Overview

"Healing is a matter of time, but it is sometimes also a matter of opportunity."

- Hippocrates

While browsing the shelves of a local bookstore or checking out top sellers online, it's obvious we are inundated with choices when it comes to the latest releases on dieting, fitness and self-help books. All claiming to have reinvented the wheel with their drastic new approach, which will no doubt have been forgotten about by next month.

So what gives? Why do these books sell so many copies, yet yield so few results for the people who buy them?

The truth of the matter is people want to live a healthier life, and they want it now. Not next week, or next month, they want it to happen right this instant, with as little effort or inconvenience as possible. Instant gratification is so prevalent these days that we pretty much expect it in all areas of life. Consumers have lost all patience, meaning that businesses and services who fail to meet these expectations are continually under the threat of sales being lost and taken elsewhere. This caused companies such as Amazon to implement same day delivery, and even Starbucks have opened drive-thru takeaways. We now live in a world where utmost convenience has become a priority, and where innovation along with success often directly relates to the speed at which an expected result is delivered, regardless of the cost or effect it has on our society.

But while most things in life can be streamlined or made easier, the one area where there are no shortcuts is our health. One of the main issues at hand is with how busy and stressful our lives have become, we tend to ignore the damage being done until it is too late. We don't have any concern for the negative consequences of our actions and our health continually takes a back seat to life's other challenges. To make matters worse, on the rare occasions we do recognise we should be adapting to healthy changes, the impulse to do something about it is often put off until later, or even dismissed. Just think, how many times have you heard someone say that from Monday they will start eating healthier or finally get some exercise? Yet when Monday arrives there is always another excuse, temptation or reason to justify not going through with it. It's probably fair to say this is something that in one way or another everyone is guilty of. In fact, I'd be lying if I said I hadn't done it countless times myself, and I'm willing to bet you have too.

People spend years neglecting and damaging their bodies and can't expect to undo the consequences overnight. Yet they do, and are willing to pay for any glimpse of hope that suggests they can do it as quickly and with as little effort as possible, so they can get straight back to their excessive lifestyle. That's why all these 'shortcut' quick fix books sell, and why publishers continue to release them. Essentially there's a constant stream of people lining up to funnel more money into a booming multibillion-dollar a year industry, and from a 'what's best for business' standpoint, why wouldn't clever marketing campaigns take full advantage of exploiting them?

In the grand scheme of things, losing weight is easy. The hard part is keeping it off in a healthy and sustainable way. But it's only difficult because of the approaches people tend to take. Studies indicate the average person trying to lose weight goes on a diet four to five times a year, inevitably quitting said diet four to five times each year. Which is evidence in itself that these approaches simply don't work and in order to finally be successful, a very different process is needed.

Part of the problem is people sabotage their progress by trying to cut out foods, which is by far the biggest issue mentally with restrictive dieting. This is because basic psychology dictates that telling yourself you can't have something simply makes you want it more, and this is exactly why these types of diets don't work. Instead all they do is continually spur on negative relationships with food, which tends to always end in an eventual binge, causing people to plummet deeper into a spiral of guilt, self-doubt and despair. This is exactly why it's essential to find a balance that keeps you sane, where you don't have to continuously place yourself under unnecessary pressure, or make life any more difficult than it needs to be.

This is one of the reasons why I personally don't believe in diets. To me, a diet represents a short-term drastic change looking for quick results, whereas what we need is a long-term sustainable lifestyle that optimises health and longevity. The way you eat needs to consist of foods you love and enjoy, where you look forward to meals and nourishing your body, not just simply being something you put up with. At the end of the day it's all about flexibility and consistency, where you regularly make positive choices that over time will help you reach your goals. In order to achieve this, it's important you are able to take a more knowledgeable approach, as that will be the only way to make more informed decisions in all aspects of your life. I have found one of the biggest keys to success is to stop dieting and start mindfully eating instead, which comes as a direct knock-on effect of these better decisions. By moving from a diet based largely around processed foods to one that focuses primarily on wholefood sources, you will be able to stop counting calories and restricting foods, stop obsessing over what you eat, and become healthier on both a mental and physical level. This has been the key factor in the people I've worked with who have been successful in not only losing weight, but also in keeping it off.

If that all sounds too simple or too good to be true, then surely with all the new approaches and 'ground breaking' ideas out there, in theory, we should be healthier than ever? But the reality is that couldn't be farther from the truth. Our world is in the midst of an epidemic, and many of the diseases plaguing society could essentially be prevented, treated or even reversed through the use of proper nutrition and lifestyle changes. Diet is however only a part of the problem, as health is influenced by everything from stress to social factors, activity levels and the ability to cope with your surrounding environment.

This is why change is needed now more than ever. Not just in the way you eat, but also in how you think, act and live. I honestly believe that in order to live a maintainable healthy lifestyle, several things need to be understood. These include what epidemics face society, how to put together a balanced diet, the problems with ever-increasing levels of stress and inactivity, and why your habits and decisions have such a negative impact on how you feel, which is exactly why all of these factors will be covered in the following chapters.

For the first time in history we live in a world where kids are expected to live shorter lives than their parents and if that doesn't scare you, it should, as you can no longer afford to be ignorant to the consequences of your actions.

"Your health is a blessing against the ailment, many passed away due to it, and some are stressed with it, live for them too, you would learn the sweetness of health."

- Qamrul Khanson

What now?

Right from the start I want you to get into the mindset that this is all about sustainable change. You have probably noticed that word was used several times in this section, but sustainability is truly what this is all about.

I want you to remember that this is not a diet. Instead, it's a lifestyle that can be designed entirely around the way you want to live your life, based on what's important to you. No, it won't happen overnight, but it will give you techniques you can apply for the rest of your life and not just to get ready for your next holiday or family event. By accepting this way of thinking now you will be able to remove a huge amount of pressure that's often attached to dieting or the idea of change, making it far easier and more enjoyable to adapt to.

I would however be lying if I said there isn't a strong element of change within this book, but the truth is, there needs to be. You can't keep eating and living the way you do and expect to lead a healthy fulfilling life, without any consequences for your actions. There's no denying that changing the way you live, think and eat will vastly improve your health, and luckily the fact that you are reading this book right now suggests you have accepted this is something you need to do. Even so, for any of this to be sustainable you need to find a way to shift your mindset from thinking this is something you must to do, to genuinely believing it's something you want and need to do. But with that in mind, the extent of how much you want to change will be your decision, as this process has been designed in a way that puts you in complete control. What differentiates this programme from others is that rather than looking to overhaul everything at once, you will be doing it at a slow and steady pace, which won't be overwhelming and you can actually enjoy as you see yourself continually progressing to better health.

That's why I definitely won't be telling you what you can and can't do. Those approaches never work and people rarely stick to them. I will however lead by example and lay out suggestions, guidance and help every step of the way, giving you the tools to self-evaluate areas of your life that need improving, along with providing guidance on how to implement this change. Your choices define who you are and whether you are not just healthy, but also happy. For some people, simply finding ways to be more active or adding more fruit and vegetables to build a more balanced diet will be a significant improvement and therefore a sufficient enough change. For others, they may have reached a point where a complete overhaul of their lifestyle and habits might be what's needed to save their health. My hope is that the information in this book will help you realise what's truly important to you. And as you progress, you will open up to a whole new world, develop new passions and interests, as well as find comfort and reward in areas you could never have previously imagined.

Activities

As you make your way through this book there will also be some activities to do that are used to highlight your goals, current habits and behaviours. These play an essential role in the final section, where they will be used to determine exactly how you need to approach the changes you will make. This is the only way to tailor this process around you and because of that they are genuinely there for a reason, and not just to fill some space. Just like anything else in life, you will get out of this process what you put into it, which is why I highly recommend that you set aside some time to complete them honestly and thoroughly, and don't just brush them off as an unimportant aspect you can skip or don't feel the need to do.

In order to help you successfully complete them and keep them together I have created an activities pack you can download for free at:

www.tailoredlifestyles.co.uk/activities

So before going any further you should print them off, as that way you have them on hand as and when they are needed.

"Health is a state of complete physical, mental and social well-being, and not merely the absence of disease or infirmity."
- **World Health Organization**

What is a healthy lifestyle?

If you look at the bigger picture, a healthy lifestyle can be broken up into four key areas, or what I like to think of as the 'four pillars' to better health.

1) Mindset and habits
2) Exercise
3) Sleep, rest and recovery
4) Diet and nutrition

The reason why I like to use the pillar concept is it makes it easy to mentally picture how it's all held together, as at the end of the day, it's all about balance. Achieving this in all areas helps to keep everything stable, whereas if one of the pillars is weak or falls down, then it puts the entire structure at risk of collapsing.

This is where so many people go wrong, as focusing on only one of these factors and ignoring the others is like trying to pull open a door that needs to be pushed. But what they don't realise is that all four areas have a direct influence on each other, and because of that, progressing in one area directly impacts the others.

For instance, improving your diet provides more energy for exercise and day-to-day activities, improves your mood, energy levels and focus, as well as aiding in sleep and recovery.

It's like a domino effect. If you start progressing in one area, then it will directly spill over into the others. Focus on all four, and you will feel better than you ever have before. On the flip side, neglecting one or more of these areas could be hugely detrimental to the rest. For example, no matter how much you exercise or how well you eat, you will never see the long term results you desire or feel the full benefit from these changes if you completely disregard rest and recovery, or fail to find ways to manage your stress levels.

It's truly worrying that researchers are finding correlations between the chronic illnesses spreading throughout our society and the growing trend of people who neglect all four aspects of what constitutes a healthy lifestyle. With some people seeming to have an almost complete disregard for proper diet and nutrition, all while engaging in little to no physical activity, getting a minimal amount of sleep and topped off with an overwhelmingly negative mindset. Findings suggest this negligence can reduce life expectancy by up to 14 years! So it really is no exaggeration to say that this is a life or death situation.

What you need to realise is that one single variable is not the problem, and that the key to better health is proper balance and not just your diet. A healthy lifestyle should be an ongoing mindset, not a gruelling punishment with an end date. That's why you should be focusing on your lifestyle as a whole instead, making sustainable changes with the overall goal being to improve your wellbeing, not starving yourself for short periods in a frail attempt to shed a few pounds. The truth is there will never be a 'right' time to focus on your wellbeing, but like with anything else in life, we tend to make time for the things we want and need. That's exactly why you need to start treating your health as a priority, rather than something that can be endlessly abused and neglected.

"Health is not simply the absence of sickness."
- Hannah Green

What are we going to be covering?

The following chapters will be looking at the epidemic we are currently facing on a global scale, along with the influence our mindset, activity levels, recovery and diet have on our overall health, and how these areas can be improved. After that we will move onto covering the basics of nutrition, how to put together a balanced diet, developing new habits, along with looking at how to integrate them into your life. By the end of this book you will not only know exactly how to put it all together, but most importantly, why you are doing it. So I make no apologies for the long-winded approach I have taken before getting to the overall point. Believe me when I say it's all for a reason. Sure, I could have just released a book with a diet and fitness plan, told you to follow it and made a quick buck. But my goal was to do something different, to help educate, guide and inspire, to change and improve your life for the better, and I honestly believe that's exactly what this will achieve.

If you are having doubts, that's fine, it's completely understandable. But what I want you to think about and remember is how obvious it is that conventional approaches aren't working. They didn't work for me and they haven't worked for you, otherwise you wouldn't be reading this now. I honestly believe this is due to not enough focus on why we are doing it. The "why" of losing weight just isn't enough, instead you need to fully understand the benefits of changing your life and the risks involved with failing to do so. While it may not be what you expect, all I ask is that you give it a chance. By the time you get to the end, you will see exactly why everything covered was so important and you will be able to make more informed decisions in all aspects of your life.

But before you go any further, I want you to make a decision. A decision that you will no longer live a life where your health takes control of you. A decision that you will open your mind to a world of possibilities where you no longer feel held down or that you have to spend your days feeling trapped or in a rut. A decision where you will do whatever it takes to actively focus on improving all four aspects that contribute towards your wellbeing. A decision that you can and will do this, that you won't give up when times get tough or when life doesn't go your way. You will push your comfort zones, take risks and embrace your journey every step of the way, because you truly are capable of amazing things.

If you can promise me that, then I promise you that together we can take back your health and you will become the best version of yourself.

With all that being said, let's begin.

The current epidemic

"The doctor of the future will no longer treat the human frame with drugs,
but rather, will cure and prevent disease with nutrition."

- Thomas Edison

While Edison may have been right with his theories on the importance of proper diet and nutrition, he couldn't have been more wrong about its perceived importance in the modern day.

The reality is that we are in the midst of an epidemic, facing catastrophe on a global scale, that in all honesty, we have in many ways brought upon ourselves. Obesity rates are at an all-time high, and we are being plagued by chronic diseases, coupled with a society filled with people who are so stressed and overwhelmed, that they are barely managing to cope. Many of these problems could and should have been avoided, but instead, they are pushing us towards the point of no return, not only with regards to our health, but our economies and environment as well.

In case you are wondering, obesity is the medical term used to describe someone who weighs at least 20 percent more than what's deemed normal for their height. Obesity now affects 24.9 percent of people in the UK, 33.5 percent in America and roughly 2.1 billion people globally, which is around 30 percent of the world's population! This is a staggering increase from the 875 million people considered obese back in 1980. These statistics become even more alarming when overweight people are thrown into the mix. Raising the numbers to 67 percent of men, and 57 percent of women in the UK now weighing more than what's considered a healthy weight. It doesn't just stop there though, as the number of overweight children has risen from one in 20, to one in five!

Another way of classifying weight is by looking at a person's BMI, with under 18.5 seen as underweight, 18.5 to 25 normal, 25 to 29.9 overweight, 30+ obese, 35+ very obese and 40+ as morbidly obese. Studies have also shown that once a person develops a BMI of over 25, they start to show signs of LDL (bad cholesterol), along with higher blood sugar levels. These symptoms and the influence they have on a person's health unsurprisingly continue to get worse the higher up the scale they go, making them more susceptible to the various illnesses we will be discussing throughout.

Obesity isn't only detrimental to individual lives, as it also places a huge financial drain on a country's economy, currently costing the UK around £47bn a year, and close to $210bn a year in America. In fact, 75 percent of health care costs in the States are spent on the maintenance or treatment of chronic diseases, many of which are directly or indirectly caused by obesity. It's pretty clear to see that as the epidemic spreads, it's set to devastate the economies of countries throughout the Western world.

It's shocking to think that we have now reached a point where more people die from obesity than starvation, which is evidence in itself of how truly skewed things have become. But if the issue at hand wasn't bad enough, I think it's fair to say that people's priorities have simply been turned upside down. No matter how you look at it, there's a fundamental flaw in society when the problem becomes mainstream entertainment and treated as a joke, rather than giving those who are affected the help and support they need. Primetime viewing is filled with shows like 'The Biggest Loser', where contestants' problems and tragedies are glorified and used for a quick laugh, rather than seeing obesity for what it truly is: a disease and an addiction, that needs to be treated just like anything else that falls into that category.

Obesity isn't the only problem either, and if anything it's merely the catalyst that spurs on other issues. In the UK, one in 17 people have been diagnosed with diabetes, and in America the rate is even higher at 9.8 percent of the population, with estimates that 27.8 percent of those are undiagnosed. In fact, every two minutes someone finds out they have diabetes, a condition that leads to 540 strokes over 140 amputations every week in the UK. All of this is made even worse when you consider that 70 percent of type 2 diabetes could be prevented or delayed by adopting a healthier diet and lifestyle. Type 2 diabetes is also an issue which used to be unheard of in children, but is now becoming a wide-spread epidemic, meaning it's undeniable that we have an obligation to our children and our children's children to stop ignoring the issues, before it's too late.

As you can no doubt guess from these statistics, chronic diseases will be a focal point popping up throughout this book. So just to clarify what I mean, the U.S. Center for Disease Control and Prevention defines chronic disease as illnesses which are not contagious and include but are not limited to: diabetes, heart disease, hypertension (high blood pressure), strokes and some forms of cancer, referring to them as "among the most common, costly and preventable of all health problems". These issues cause seven out of ten deaths every year, and affect the lives of 113 million Americans, which is almost half of the adult population! The European Association for the Study of Obesity has released figures showing that 2.8 million deaths per year are a direct result of being overweight or obese. On top of that more than 40 million children under the age of five are now overweight, with these figures on the rise every year.

To make matters worse, roughly 20 percent of people who lose their lives every year die from illnesses caused by their dietary and lifestyle choices.

Just let that sink in for a moment.

That's one in five deaths every year, that could have possibly been prevented. The famous saying of 'one death is a tragedy, a million is a statistic' seems more shockingly apparent than ever. Except now it's not due to war, famine or genocide, but instead is simply down to poor dietary and lifestyles choices, stress and a lack of physical activity.

With chronic diseases and obesity affecting more and more people every day, it leaves the simple question, what's going wrong?

Over the last 100 years our modern diet has drastically changed. Foods are now more processed and refined, as people have become addicted to salty, fatty, fried and sugary options, eating food-like products instead of actual food. Eating like this has escalated to the point where 70 percent of the American diet now comes from processed foods that have been so heavily modified, that they are almost unrecognisable from their original form. Other countries in the Western world are quickly following this trend, which is why it's no surprise that obesity rates are highest in developed countries. But, as with everything else in our world, these problems are spreading further afield, as globalisation is allowing people in third world countries to gain access to the products and services at the heart of the issue.

Obesity and disease aren't the only problems either, as further research has shown the Western diet of sugary snacks, takeaways, pre-packaged meals and processed meats leads to higher rates of depression, anxiety and stress. These foods may even be linked to mental disorders such as Alzheimers, Schizophrenia, ADHD and some studies have even suggested a diet revolving around these products has caused an increase in suicide among young people.

The Western world has an innate reaction to panic whenever there's a perceived threat towards them or their safety. A prime example being the Ebola 'epidemic' causing what for many, can only be described as a complete meltdown. The news portrayed it like it was the end of the world, with people fearing for their lives, cancelling trips, avoiding certain foods and refusing to go out in public, when in fact, the direct danger was nearly non-existent. Yet at present we are in the middle of an epidemic that's actually a direct tangible threat, and people seem to be taking no notice. With one in five people literally killing themselves because they aren't eating properly or are making negligent lifestyle choices. Nothing is said or done about these habits that are bringing endless pain and misery to millions, as somehow everything is just swept under the rug. On paper it seems like such a ridiculous problem to be having. It almost sounds like a fictional story, or something that is so far-fetched it couldn't possibly be true. After all, that couldn't actually be happening...could it? But the sad truth is, we live in a world where people are literally eating and abusing their bodies to death, and suffering every step of the way.

"Time and health are two precious assets that we don't recognize and appreciate until they have been depleted."
- Denis Waitley

The bigger picture

I think it's fair to say that as people's lives have become more and more hectic, their priorities and mindset's have become massively out of line with what's truly important. Most people's attitudes and understanding about health and food are simply wrong, thinking they are invincible and will never get the diseases so many others are facing. Then once the inevitable happens, they wonder how it could have happened to them and blame everyone else but themselves, rather than accepting responsibility for the long-term actions that brought them there in the first place.

Part of the problem is we are continuously turning to what is convenient, looking to save a few precious minutes everywhere we can. We spend countless amounts of money and time on things we don't need, while neglecting what should be a priority for our basic survival. Without thinking, people will regularly spend money on some sugar filled choco-pumkpin-syrup-latte or fast food option. But when presented with vegetables or healthy alternatives in a supermarket, complain about the price and go for cheaper options instead, even though these fresh products are still a fraction of the cost of that takeaway lunch they bought earlier.

Another issue is the food industry itself. Throughout supermarkets consumers are bombarded and misled with false information portraying 'healthy' options, many of which are just as bad as their unhealthy counterparts. With confusing food labels, food manufacturing companies are able to continuously lie to consumers, taking full advantage of misinformation spread by fad diets and trends. This in turn means that the majority of people seem to be completely unaware of the extent to which processed products and package marketing affect their diet and therefore their lives, nor do they realise how food corporations contribute to the epidemic of obesity and its related illnesses.

Like all businesses, a food company's primary concern is to sell more products. Therefore, they have perfected misleading advertising and regularly twist the truth to manipulate people into believing their products are healthy. A prime example of this is Coca-Cola's Vitaminwater. A product originally marketed as 'an excellent source of nutrition', that could be used as a healthy alternative to soda. It was promoted using outlandish claims that it provided essential nutrients, was filled with antioxidants and could boost immunity. Yet upon proper investigation, it was found to be just another sugar-filled drink, with up to 31 grams of sugar per bottle and little to no added health benefits. I'd also like to highlight that this in itself is already above the recommended intake of 30 total grams of sugar per day, and this is just from one drink! Meaning there's a good chance that when consumed it will be just a fraction of your total sugar for the day.

Michael F. Jacobson, Executive Director at the non-profit advocacy group Center for Science in the Public Interest stated, "Vitaminwater, like Coca-Cola itself, promotes weight gain, obesity, diabetes, heart disease and cannot deliver on any of the dishonest claims it has made over the years". In fact, research conducted by the University of Berkley in California suggests that between 1977 and 2007 at least 20 percent of America's weight gain has been due to sugary drinks.

In the end, Coca-Cola was charged with a class action lawsuit and their defence pretty much came down to 'no reasonable person could be misled into thinking Vitaminwater was a "healthy drink"'. A defence showing complete negligence and disregard for a duty of care towards their consumers and even still, it has done little to deter consumers from using the product.

What's even worse is a large proportion of studies conducted into food safety and regulations are funded by the very people in question. In scientific practice it's not uncommon for funding to be provided by the industry whose subject is being studied. Research into this matter suggests that when this is the case, findings are often unsurprisingly biased. In fact, an article in the Public Library of Science Medicine journal found that when conducting research into the sugar industry and the American Beverage Association, studies by scientists with no financial ties to big corporations were five times more likely to find a link between sugary drinks and weight gain than those funded by organisations such as Coca-Cola and PepsiCo. There have also been numerous cases where dieticians have been criticised for portraying Coke as a healthy snack in return for continued payments and funding.

Surely this is a conflict of interest and no different from a murderer being tasked with finding and presenting evidence against themselves? Of course they will find a way to portray it in a light that makes them look innocent and not guilty of causing any harm. This may seem like an extreme example, but if you actually think about it, it really isn't. The processed foods people are being fed are literally poisoning and killing them, with the diseases that develop from ingesting them simply a side effect of what's being introduced into their bodies. The companies producing these products know exactly how harmful, unhealthy and addictive they are, and still they go out of their way to ensure customers keep spending and consuming in higher and higher volumes.

However, while you can blame big businesses and their marketing campaigns all you want, ultimately everyone is responsible and accountable for their own choices and decisions. The aim of this book isn't to point fingers, play the blame game, or go into the non-existent social obligations that should be adhered to by these corporations. The above examples were simply to bring your attention to the extent in which we are misled on a daily basis and how you need to be careful about what you choose to believe. The reality of the matter is that the corporations in question are simply there to fulfil a supply because there is a demand. Unfortunately, the demand is there for the products causing so many health problems in our society, rather than those mentioned earlier: unprocessed wholefoods. It's because of this that real progress will never be made until there are fundamental changes to the wants and needs within society.

"Illness or disease is only Nature's warning that filth has accumulated in some portion or other of the body; and it would surely be the part of wisdom to allow Nature to remove the filth, instead of covering it up with the help of medicines."
- **Mahatma Gandhi**

The issue at hand

It's not that people don't want to be healthy. Everywhere you look these days we are being sold on some new product or service to improve our lives. Billions are spent every year on the latest diet and fitness trends, but this is a problem in itself, as people are making drastic but temporary changes, looking for a quick fix or miracle results. This month it may be low fat, next month it will be low carb, and marketers will continue to spin the same ideas in different ways until you buy into the concept that they finally got it right. Except they won't have and all that will happen is people will continue to jump from one diet to another, until the day when they either give up and simply accept the way things are, or finally realise the errors they have been making all along.

If you need further convincing, then the University of Los Angeles California found that 'up to two thirds of those on a diet regain more weight than when they started'. So yes, while you can lose weight with these approaches, it's rarely maintainable, as people simply revert back to their old ways upon completion.

Looking closer at the bigger picture shows us that we have a population constantly indulging for momentary satisfaction, eating thousands of excess calories everyday, yet placing themselves in a state where they are nutritionally starving. Time and time again it's been said that 'food is the most abused anxiety drug and exercise is the most under-utilised antidepressant', yet time and time again this advice is ignored.

I know this opening section has largely focused on food, but that's because it's such a huge part of the puzzle. It's been proven that proper nutrition can prevent, treat or in some cases even reverse chronic diseases and this is all achievable through fundamental lifestyle changes.

What it all comes down to is this: you need to ask yourself, what's more important than the health of you and your family? It could easily be argued that an investment in your health is the most important investment you could ever make, especially when considering that studies suggest that 70 percent of the illnesses making up this epidemic are brought about by lifestyle choices people make, such as smoking, drinking, bad diet and lack of exercise. The other 30 percent is based on luck and genetics.

Sure, there's no guarantee, but isn't it better to reduce the odds and stack the deck in your favour? Rather than actively escalating them?

I know this chapter has gone on a bit and bounced from point to point, but luckily though it's not all doom and gloom. All this change is achievable. The point of this section was to raise your awareness about the extent of the epidemic we are facing, get you thinking about how all these things are related, and the risks of continuing down the path of such a negligent lifestyle. Hopefully this will have helped you realise why changing the way you live and act is so important. Not only are you putting your own health at risk, but society, the economy and the planet are also being heavily impacted. I know it's a lot to process and take in. A few years ago I was in the exact same situation as you, completely unaware of how bad things truly were and oblivious to the impact of my actions. If this all comes as a bit of a shock or reality check for you don't worry, as you certainly aren't alone. If anything, you are in the majority. As daunting as this may all seem, or as much as you may believe it's impossible for you to achieve, you can and will make the transition into a healthier, more fulfilling lifestyle.

That's why the focus is going to be shifted back to you and we are going to break up the elements that influence your wellbeing, looking at them one at a time, along with how they can be improved.

Before we move on, just a quick reminder of the sections we will be covering:

1) Mindset and habits
2) Exercise
3) Sleep, rest and recovery
4) Diet and nutrition

By now you should be starting to see how all the aspects impacting your wellbeing are related, and why they are so important. Once we have looked at them all individually, we will then look at how to put together a plan that's completely tailored around your personal journey.

"Man is not what he thinks he is, he is what he hides."

- André Malraux

Activity 1

Keeping a food diary

Later on we will be looking at how to put together a balanced diet, but before getting to that, it's important you get an idea of how and what you currently eat. This will be the only way to get a complete understanding of the choices you are making and see where you could benefit most from making changes. Not only that, but incorporating this activity now as you work your way through this book has the added bonus of getting you to become more mindful and self-aware of your actions and behaviours, which in turn will directly spill over into other areas as well.

The problem is that many people have a far higher calorie intake than they realise, as they often forget to consider that occasional biscuit or chocolate, which in many cases could be a daily, or even multiple times a day occurrence. This is commonly referred to as 'secret eating', as often the person involved doesn't even realise they are doing it, as it's merely out of habit or a response to deal with emotions or other feelings such as stress or boredom. These instances can have a dramatic influence on your overall progress, as they quickly add up and often explains why people have such a hard time losing weight. This is usually one of the first practices I get all my new clients to complete and most of them often come back with a shocked realisation of not only what they are actually eating, but also how much. It really is an eye opening activity, as with how busy life is it's easy to get lost in the motions and completely disregard what you are actually doing.

That's why for the next week I want you to keep a food diary of everything you eat, making a note of what the meal consisted of and the time in which you ate it. Include any drinks that aren't water, along with anything added to them, such as milk or sugar.

On top of showing what you consumed, by keeping a food diary you will also be able to determine if there are certain cues or situations where you are regularly making bad choices. For instance, maybe everyday you take an afternoon trip to the vending machine, turn to sugar after a stressful meeting, or even have cake every time you see a certain friend.

What you need to do

This really needs to be an honest reflection of how you regularly eat, so for the next week I want you to eat exactly the same way as you normally would, without changing anything at all. Along with the meals or snacks you have, it's also helpful to state how you were feeling at the time, as that way you can look for connections between negative emotions and decisions. If you want to take it a step further, you can even score your hunger level between one to ten at each meal, as this will give you a better idea as to whether you are eating out of hunger, or simply out of habit because there's food available.

This is the easiest way to learn to start listening to your body and recognising the signs it's giving you. How you choose to record it is up to you, but make sure you do it as and when you consume something. This is absolutely essential, because at the end of the day it's often difficult to recall exactly what you ate, meaning items can easily be missed off or forgotten and in many cases these will usually be the high calorie in the moment snacks.

The easiest way to do this is to make a note on your phone every time you have something, including the time, date and what it was. Alternatively, you could carry a small notebook around, or even take pictures of your meals on your phone.

Choose whichever method works best for you and at the end of each day or week, enter the information into the food diary tables, which can be found in the downloadable activities pack over at:

www.tailoredlifestyles.co.uk/activities

An example of what the tables look like can be seen below:

Time	Food/drink	Comments	Hunger level

Once you have completed your food diary make sure you look after it, as it will be a vital tool in the putting it all together section and play a massive role later on in this process.

Pillar One

Mindset and Habits

"To me, good health is more than just exercise and diet. It's really a point of view and a mental attitude you have about yourself."
- Albert Schweitzer

While everything discussed within this book is important for a healthy lifestyle, our mindset is very much what brings it all together, playing a fundamental role in everything from our behaviour, to our actions, thoughts, emotions, beliefs, and decisions. It has long been theorised that there exists a 'mind-body connection', linking our mindset with our physical health, and for the first time in the 1970s, strong evidence was documented in support of this belief. Many people believe the mind-body connection only works on a mundane level, where if you have a more positive outlook and feel better about yourself, you are more likely to take steps towards looking after your health. Research however has found it to go far deeper than that, finding direct hard-wired connections in the form of nerve pathways in the central nervous system, leading from the brain, to the cells in the immune system. It has been documented that on the surface of the immune system there are receptors which act like key holes for the brains chemical neurotransmitters, and during times of stress, your brain's response is to release these neurotransmitters, which then affect the cells in your immune system. The opposite can happen as well, as chemicals released by your immune system can directly affect your brain.

To simplify this and give you a better idea of it in action, have you ever noticed how tired and fatigued you feel when you are sick? This is simply due to how much energy your immune system requires when fighting illnesses, as your body is forced to prioritises one function over the rest, as it needs to deal with the immediate attack. This is your immune system affecting how your brain functions, and if you are constantly stressed and overwhelmed, you are continuously placing your body in this strenuous state. This goes a long way in explaining why people with a grim outlook on life are often tired or low on energy, as their bodies are always fighting an internal battle, where it's a vicious cycle of feeling down, but not having the energy or power to change it.

In many ways, our mindset is our belief about ourselves and our most basic qualities. For instance, think about your personality, intelligence and talents. Are these set in stone? Or are they aspects you can change, grow and develop throughout your life? People who are fixed in their mindset believe that nothing can change the way things are, causing them to worry about these traits and how adequate they are, causing self-doubt and a belief that they aren't good enough. This in turn can directly spill over into all areas of their lives, affecting not only how they think or act, but also how their body responds.

For many of us a negative mindset is simply something we bring upon ourselves, as we create feelings of negativity and doubt, unable to objectively separate the meaning in circumstances from reality. For those of us trapped in this way of thinking, at some point in our lives something happened to make us believe that this is who we are and what we deserve. This state of mind causes us to blame everyone else for our problems, when at the very core, it is our self-belief that is the issue, and we hide behind these barriers not wanting to face the truth. It is only when we accept this, that we can finally overcome them and start to change.

We have all faced adversity in our lives, and been in situations that have changed who we are as people, along with how we think and behave. Often these situations may have left behind numerous scars we hold onto, but the only way to move forward is to let them go. Just because someone said or made you feel a certain way, doesn't make it real. When you accept this it will sink in and have a domino effect on other areas of your life, and you will be able to move forward and progress, rather than holding yourself back.

Part of the problem with our state of mind is that we become so fixated on the end result in everything that we do, that we forget to live and enjoy the present. Even though at times it may not seem like it, you do have a choice with everything you do, and you need to make a choice to stop just being present. Anything you have ever done, felt, said or experienced is in the past and you can't change it, but what you can do is focus on now. Stop thinking 'I'm going to be happy when this happens'. You can and need to choose to be happy now.

A negative mindset isn't just caused by past feelings or emotions, and it can also be brought on by the challenges and strains we face everyday. After all, our world has evolved in such a way that we are under a tremendous amount of pressure, constantly stressed, and regularly having to prioritise everything else above ourselves. It's no surprise that this inevitably takes its toll on our mental health, pushing us into a state of mind where we feel overwhelmed to the point of waiting for it all to fall apart. This spurs on negative thoughts and emotions, pushing us into a rut from which it's difficult to escape. From time to time it's only natural to get drawn into this way of thinking; that's just human nature. Part of the problem was discovered by Stanford University, who estimates that as much as 90 percent of our thoughts are actually repetitive. This makes it highly problematic for people who have a negative mindset, as they become stuck thinking the same detrimental thoughts over and over. This means repetitive thinking is not only an issue in relation to general happiness, but it can also influence our health if we feel trapped, stressed and overwhelmed. For this reason, it's absolutely essential to recognise when or if you are repetitively thinking negative thoughts, as becoming aware is an essential part of breaking free and actively making changes.

Our mindset can also be heavily shaped and influenced by the people around us, meaning that if we are constantly surrounded by negativity, we are more likely to be negative ourselves. Not only that, but we tend to behave in a way that adheres to societal norms, often acting in a manner that we believe is expected of us, regardless as to whether or not it is who we are or what we want.

My favourite example of this in action is a story about how a group of scientists took five monkeys and placed them in a cage, with a ladder in the middle and bananas at the top of it. Whenever a monkey started to climb the ladder, the rest of the monkeys were soaked with cold water. Eventually every time a monkey would attempt to climb the ladder, the rest would pull it off and beat it up. After a while no monkey dared to even try, regardless of the temptation. The scientists then replaced one of the monkeys, who immediately tried to start climbing the ladder, only to be pulled off and beaten up by the rest of the group, unaware of why this was happening. After the monkey received several beatings, it learned to never try climbing the ladder, even though there was no reason not to, apart from the beatings. Following this, a second monkey was substituted, and the same pattern followed, only this time the first monkey participated in delivering the beatings. Then a third monkey was changed and the process repeated, followed by a fourth, until finally the fifth was replaced as well.

What the scientists now had was a group of monkeys, who without ever having received a cold shower, would continue to beat up any other monkey who tried to climb the ladder. If we were able to ask the monkeys why they were beating up those who attempted to climb the ladder, in all likelihood their answer would be 'I don't know, that's just what's done around here'.

I think this story applies perfectly to everyday life, as we behave in a way that we are scared to take control or try anything new, and we react in manners we don't fully understand or comprehend. This places us in a state that psychology teachings have named "the learned helplessness syndrome", where repeatedly being placed in situations where we feel helpless or unable to escape can cause our direct response to be giving up trying. This lack of control means an inability to make a positive change or influence an outcome, which in turn deters mental health and causes further emotional damage. These thoughts are common in the workplace, where often procedures are fixed, making little room for personal growth or change. This rigid environment can then engulf other areas of our lives, as we get so used to being compliant, that we no longer even question why things are the way they are. This can make us grow used to conditions, including everything from depression to anxiety, making them not so much of a biological issue, but more of a mental one. So when it comes to tackling the issues you face and outcomes you want to achieve, initially it's not about the changes that you make, but instead is more about taking control and knowing that in fact, you do have a choice.

With all the advances in modern science, one thing has become abundantly clear – our minds have the power to heal, but at the same time they also have the power to wreak havoc on our health, mentally, physically and emotionally. That's why we need to recognise and identify the impact our thoughts and emotions have not just on each other, but also on our relationships, behaviours and body. Our brain has the first line of the connection to our bodies' defence, and the easiest way to understand how our mind can affect our body, is to look at stress.

"If you treat every situation as a life and death matter, you will die a lot of times."

- **Dean Smith**

Stress

Even though stress doesn't directly cause disease, it has been shown to speed up the development of problems that already exist in the body or brain, which is why stress has been directly linked to the majority of chronic illnesses. The more you continue to burn the candle at both ends and fail to find balance, the more you increase your risks of developing or exacerbating their growth. Studies have also shown chronic stress and negative emotions drain mental energy, upsetting the body's hormonal balance and depleting the brain of the chemicals that influence feelings of happiness. This leads to an array of health problems, from high blood pressure to headaches, loss of sleep and even digestive issues. New scientific studies have even shown chronic stress actually affects our DNA strands; shortening telomeres (DNA end caps), which directly affect the role of aging, and can even shorten our lifespan. This, in part explains why research suggests people with a positive mindset are likely to live longer, as they place less strain on their bodies, allowing it to more easily fight off disease and recover.

The basic survival reaction

Since the beginning of human existence, our body's main priority has been to defend itself against threats that could result in injury or loss of life. Through these experiences, the body learned to prioritise the bad over good. While this is ideal in a highly dangerous or volatile environment, in our modern world we are no longer roaming around in the wilderness in danger of being eaten by wild animals, placed in a position of having to find shelter, or desperately hunting or gathering to try and find food. Meaning this involuntary reaction is rarely necessary anymore.

But while our world has evolved in many ways, on a biological level our bodies still act and respond in the same way. Unfortunately, this prioritising of bad over good means people subconsciously focus too much on the minor frustrations in life, which is perpetuated by the unconscious tendency to repetitively think the same thoughts. This goes a long way in showcasing exactly why life's little frustrations can have such a profound influence on how people feel mentally and emotionally. Everything from having to queue, getting stuck in traffic, or simply not being able to find their keys, has the ability to push us over the edge.

The only way to change is by focusing on evaluating how and why it occurs, so that you can determine the cause and what's likely to set it off. Often these small setbacks are spurred on by a deeper issue, and the event itself is just what pushes people too far. It could be anything from huge pressure and stress at work, to an annoying co-worker or a nagging sound coming from the other end of the office. All day it eats away at you, building up till the traffic is the final straw that makes you snap. There's only so much you can take, as this constant frustration causes you to get burnt out on life, where often your breaking point can be triggered by something that, in isolation, would barely have bothered you.

So what can be done about it?

Making changes starts with being more mindful, which is all about noticing new things, such as ideas, people or experiences, along with thinking about our actions, and why we behave or respond the way that we do, allowing us to become more aware of our surroundings. This mental state allows us to focus our awareness on the present moment. So next time you face a difficult situation, you need to take a step back, take a deep breath and try to relax. By being aware of the triggers, you can begin to manage your stress levels and start sending the right signals to the brain. By practicing being mindful, over time, you will be able to change the way you view and interact with the world.

What many books on wellbeing will tell you is that in order to improve your health you need to reduce stress. While this is all well and good, in reality it really isn't that simple. Often, an average person will work long hours then have a nightmare of a commute home, followed by rushing around trying to look after and feed the kids, until finally hoping for some time with their partner, before getting a minimal amount of rest, just to repeat it all the next day. Therefore, telling us to reduce stress is not only unfeasible, but is also pretty useless and insulting advice, often given by someone completely out of touch with what life in the real world is actually like. What you need to be focusing on instead, is finding ways in which to manage your stress levels.

In moments of despair, or when you feel like you are being pushed a little bit further than you can stretch, there's a simple and easy-to-use technique which revolves around your breathing that I recommend trying. This exercise can do wonders for your body and mind, whether you are feeling overwhelmed, struggling with a high-pressure situation, got hit with a sudden urge of cravings, or merely need to unwind. You can apply it to any situation or circumstance where you feel discomfort, unease, or out of your comfort zone. Just to back up its reputation for effectiveness, this practice is taught to staff within the UK National Health Service to help them calm down in moments of crisis, when dealing with conflict, or other challenging situations.

The entire purpose of this exercise is to slow your heart rate, which directly enables you to think more clearly. The reason why this is so effective is it helps to settle feelings of panic, as during these times our breathing tends to speed up, causing us to take shallower breaths, which in turn reduces the amount of oxygen we take in. This can further escalate both the problem and our responses, as our brains use 25 percent of the oxygen when inhale. Because of that, reduced intake can cause problems such as difficulties concentrating or maintaining focus, and it's during these moments that we often need these abilities the most. This can lead to us making in the moment responses, where our judgement is clouded and we are simply acting on impulse. You will be amazed at how something so simple as taking a moment to get your thoughts under control can have such a big impact on your emotions and reactions.

Breathing exercise

To perform this exercise:

- Close your eyes (if possible) and take a deep breath in through your nose and out through your mouth.

- Take slow deep breaths in as you count to four, then repeat as you breath out.

- Feel your heart rate slow down and your mind relax as you keep a steady tempo.

- Don't pause or hold your breath, and if you can't do a count of four, instead do what feels comfortable.

- Focus solely on your breathing so that you can try and clear your mind, soothing any negative emotions, as you calm down in moments of elevated and aggravated stress.

- Continue until you feel calm and relaxed, ready to cope or respond more positively to the situation, then carry on with your day or what you are doing.

There's a good chance after reading these steps you are thinking it sounds silly, that there's no way it will possibly work and it definitely isn't something for you. I'll even be the first to admit that you asked me to try this a few years ago, I'd probably have laughed at you. On paper I completely get it, as I used to be that guy, dismissive of anything I viewed as weird or strange, from yoga to meditation, or any other ritual recommended for helping you relax. But they are now practices I regularly incorporate into my weekly routine, which in itself goes to show how much you can shift your mindset, so trust me and give it a go.

Practice makes perfect

One of the most common signs of a negative mindset is an individual's level of hostility, which is frequently caused by having an adverse view of life. Anger is often repressed and builds up causing them to snap over the smallest frustrations, rarely able to see the good in things and regularly overreacting to issues that in essence, are hardly a big deal. In turn, this can lead to a range of issues, from high blood pressure to cardiovascular disease, and the only way to resolve and improve what's going on in the body is to become mindful that you have overreacted, recognise why it happened, then find ways to calm down and relax. If you are prone to having issues or find yourself regularly in circumstances where you lose your cool, then it's definitely worth practicing this technique at home to get the hang of it and see how it works best for you. From this you will be able to put the action to better use in situations where it's needed, and you may even find it's exactly what you need after a long day to help you unwind. It could even be something you incorporate into your evening routine, as a way to relax before going to sleep.

Let's take a look at a everyday stressful situation, and see how this can be put into action.

There's no denying everyone hates being stuck in traffic. Personally, I find it one of the most frustrating and infuriating situations to be found in, especially after a long day when all you want to do is finally get home and relax. But like many other things in life, it's often unavoidable and nothing can be done about it unless you magically find a short cut, or invent a flying car.

Rather than get frustrated or let it get to you, focus instead on developing the mindset that acknowledges that this situation is indeed, out of your control, and because of that getting irate over it achieves nothing except to further aggravate you or ruin your day. As hard as it is, you need to consciously tell yourself to accept it for what it is and that you are not going to let it get to you. I know me telling you to not let it get to you sounds redundant or easier said than done. But by acknowledging the problem, you have admitted it's also impossible for you to change it, which means you can actively begin to work on changing the mental state associated with the issue.

Next time you are in this situation or one like it and start feeling yourself getting angry, anxious or overwhelmed with negativity, take a look out the window and appreciate your surroundings. Look at the trees and the sky, the people outside enjoying life, take slow deep breaths and ease your heart rate. People get so caught up in everyday life that they miss the wonder in the world passing by them on a daily basis. They miss it because they fail to notice the environment around them. So instead of focusing on the inconvenience of the situation, shift the focus to your breathing and appreciate the moment. By implementing this you can at least try to relax and soothe the negative energy.

Maybe your pessimistic mindset jumped straight to thinking that doesn't help when you are stuck in gridlock on the motorway with nothing around. Or maybe even that it sounds like a stupid idea? Once again, immediately trying to find fault and thinking of the bad in a proposed solution? If so, that's exactly the detrimental mindset I'm talking about that needs to be worked on and changed. So in this case, rather than getting frustrated by being stuck in the car, try to see it as an opportunity to reflect on your day, what you have to be thankful for, what you are looking forward to, a bit of "me time", or view it as some down time away from the other stress and pressure you have faced throughout the day.

Use this time to think about where you are going, what you want to achieve and how you are going to get there, turning a period of inconvenience into one for self-reflection and improvement. Your breathing is essential in these moments and the previously mentioned exercise can be used as a tool to help you ease the tension and relax. By practicing mindfulness in times of despair, you are able to not only influence how you react to stress, but also the impact the effects of stress has on your health, as you are aiding in the right kind of signals being sent from your brain, to your immune system. Another added benefit is that by recognising situations of negativity and consciously working on changing them, you not only improve your mindset and health, but people's perceptions of you as well.

Making changes might mean learning to accept the situations for what they are, finding ways to deal with them, or even changing your environment. It all comes down to your individual circumstances and how much control you can have over them, and if it's not something you can get control of, then it's all about finding ways to reduce the control and influence they have over you. Learning how you can control (or even more importantly - make use of) a stressful situation will alleviate or minimise negative thoughts. Therefore, regardless of what the trigger situations are, you will be able to find ways to improve how you cope and react in the midst of them, by becoming self-aware of your behaviour.

"It's not stress that kills us, it is our reaction to it."

- Hans Selye

The overlooked influence of hormones

Your body has miraculous healing abilities and its self-repair mechanism can do everything from kill cancer cells to fight infection and slow down how quickly you age. But it's only able to do so when the nervous system is functioning properly and not hindered as it is in times of perceived danger. The body's response during these times is to release the hormones cortisol and epinephrine, and it's often underestimated just how much of an influence they can actually have when elevated levels are released or remain in the bloodstream.

Cortisol is the body's way of reacting to situations where it deems itself as under attack, as a response mechanism to deal with the perceived threat. Epinephrine on the other hand is more commonly referred to as adrenaline, and its release can be brought on by strong emotions such as anger or fear. During instances of heightened discomfort, the body enters what's often referred to as 'fight or flight mode', where the bloodstream is flooded with glucose to act as an immediate energy source and insulin production is inhibited to prevent this glucose from being stored, favouring it instead for immediate use. While cortisol narrows the arteries, epinephrine increases the heart rate, forcing blood to pump harder and faster. At this time, functions deemed non-essential or detrimental to these circumstances are stopped or slowed down, suppressing everything from the digestive, to growth, immune and reproductive systems until the threat has passed and hormonal levels return to normal.

In small doses there's nothing harmful about these responses, and in fact, during some activities such as exercise, they can actually be beneficial in short-term bursts. However, problems begin when the body is persistently placed in this state, which unfortunately, is often the reality of the fast-paced, high pressure and stressful lifestyle so many people find themselves in every day. This aspect of your wellbeing really is a vicious circle, as a negative outlook can be linked to causing the release of cortisol, on top of actually being one of the side effects of elevated levels. This is due to how it suppresses production of the feel good hormone serotonin, which can lead to feelings of depression, along with panic, anxiety, paranoia, excessive worrying and even fear.

To put this into perspective, think about a time when you were in the build-up to a high-pressure event, such as waiting to go into an exam, a job interview, presentation or an important meeting. Remember how anxious and nervous you were? Your heart no doubt racing, stomach tightening, as you began to doubt yourself and wonder have you done enough preparation? Are you good enough? Are you going to make a fool of yourself? Is this the moment everything falls apart? Unable to think straight, panicking as nerves slowly start to get the better of you, longing for it just to be over as your mind starts focusing on worst case scenarios and what could go wrong.

There's no denying these events put a huge strain on your body, now imagine doing that to yourself each and every day. Sounds horrible doesn't it? That's exactly what people are doing without even realising it, when they let chronic stress and a negative mindset gain a foothold in their life. Everyday they burden their body with these emotions, and continuously being pushed out of their comfort zones causes a roller-coaster ride of entering fight or flight mode, which the body is simply unable to effectively adapt or respond to.

Stress is a huge trigger for the release of cortisol, which in turn can build up and cause depression, anxiety, insomnia and weight gain, due to a reduced sensitivity to insulin, with long-term effects including everything from fatigue to fertility problems, thyroid disorders and dementia. When in this state, the body is constantly dealing with the strain of high blood pressure and fluctuating insulin levels. This is partly why increased cortisol levels elevate the risk of developing chronic diseases such as diabetes, hypertension and heart disease.

As you can see, stress isn't the only problem, and constant negativity can also lead to depression, an illness Dr. Michael Frenneaux, the professor of cardiovascular medicine at the University of Birmingham, suggests can double the risk of a heart attack in an otherwise healthy person. Furthermore, research suggests that the process of cortisol release causes damage to arteries, which explains the direct link between stress and cardiovascular disease.

Cortisol levels aren't just increased by stress though, as they can also be brought on by feelings of sadness, worry, exhaustion, anxiety, or even over exercising. To make matters worse, the gastrointestinal system can also be impacted, as it's highly sensitive to these hormones, especially at elevated levels. This can lead to a wide array of problems from heartburn to nausea, constipation, diarrhoea or even abdominal cramps. You may have noticed stress is linked to sudden sugar cravings, which are brought on by rapid swings in blood sugar levels, which in turn can be caused by cortisol due to how it influences your response to insulin. This explains those moments of stress eating, searching for a sugar hit or food that gives you a perceived feeling of temporary comfort, which is why numerous studies have linked cortisol to weight gain and excessive eating.

A real world example

There was a time when I was really stressed with everything from work to general life, on a highly restrictive diet, in a calorie deficit and training really hard in the gym trying to lose weight. I remember feeling under constant pressure, like I was trapped and sinking, with no way out in sight. Everyday was a constant struggle just to get by, with the consequences of all these issues causing my cortisol levels to go through the roof. Because of that not only did I get severe insomnia where I struggled to sleep, I was also moody, exhausted, had no energy, constantly negative and had a substantial drop in testosterone.

My decisions and lifestyle placed a huge strain on my body and it reacted accordingly, and it's only now looking back that I realise the huge and adverse effect it had on my wellbeing. At the time I was almost blinded to the fact that it was happening, as I was so mentally, physically and emotionally drained, that I was just trying to get through the day. My relationships with my family were strained, I was struggling with work, neglecting responsibilities and what little rest I did get involved hours of lying in bed trying to fall asleep, followed by waking up pretty much every hour throughout the night. It's fair to say I wasn't in a good place and as you can see it's an understatement to say that failure to find balance in an all-or-nothing approach had a huge influence on my health, mindset and outlook. I wasn't alone in feeling this way either, as it's a constant state so many others find themselves in each day. The biggest issue with all this is that often we can be completely unaware of what we are facing, or the extent in which stress is truly influencing our behaviour, making us feel trapped, helpless, and unlikely to find a way out.

"We can easily manage if we will only take, each day, the burden appointed to it. But the load will be too heavy for us if we carry yesterday's burden over again today, and then add the burden of the morrow before we are required to bear it."

- John Newton

Reducing stress hormones

If you recognise you are suffering from any of these symptoms or living in similar conditions from what you have read so far, then it's highly likely your cortisol levels are elevated and the only way you will take back your health is to actively focus on decreasing them.

I'm not going to lie, lowering both your stress and cortisol levels will take time, requiring a large amount of consistency, focus and dedication. Personally, it took me several months to get them under control, but with some lifestyle changes, it is possible to return them to a more normal level. If you are really struggling it may even be worth visiting a doctor and getting him or her to run some tests to see exactly where your levels are at and how your body is responding.

In order to decrease your levels, you need to recognise the factors that contribute towards them becoming elevated in the first place, and then find ways to implement the changes listed below to achieve some sort of balance and control. You will see all these changes discussed in detail at various points throughout this book, as they all play integral role in developing a healthier lifestyle.

These changes include:

- Finding ways to minimise or manage stress.

- Adapting to a diet based primarily around wholefoods, with a low glycaemic load.

- Eating more vegetables, fruits, whole grains, nuts, beans and seeds to increase your intake of fibre, antioxidants and phytonutrients (nutrients found in certain plants beneficial towards health).

- Making sure you have no deficiencies in your diet and meet your required intake levels for Omega-3 fatty acids.

- Finding ways to be less sedentary and more active.

- If you are over training/exercising too much, look to give your body a break to properly recover.

- Aim to get six to eight hours sleep a night.

- Ensure you find ways to relax and clear your mind.

- Reduce your consumption of alcohol, caffeine, sugar and processed foods.

With the ever-growing rates of chronic diseases, it's becoming increasingly apparent that more and more people are reaching the stage where illnesses are simply a side effect caused by prioritising everything else above their wellbeing. Therefore, a balanced healthy lifestyle begins when you start taking responsibility for your own wellbeing, as no one else is going to do it for you. That's why you need to realise it's ok to say no at times and that occasionally, you need to take a step back, relax and take charge to prioritise yourself.

Because at the end of the day, without your health, what do you truly have?

You often hear of people landing up in hospital with life-changing illnesses, saying they wish they had done it all differently. Wishing they hadn't worked so many hours, made more time for their family and friends, took that long overdue trip, or simply appreciated what life has to offer. Praying that if given the opportunity they will completely change who they are and start showing appreciation for what they have. My dad was a prime example, lying in a hospital bed close to death, saying it took all of that to happen for him to realise how much he had taken life and what he had for granted.

But that doesn't have to be you. You can start making changes now before it is too late, before you get to that moment of forced realisation and wonder how you got it so wrong.

"When I look back on all these worries, I remember the story of the old man who said on his deathbed that he had had a lot of trouble in his life, most of which had never happened."

- Winston Churchill

A more positive mindset

There's no two ways around it. The simple truth is that people who have a more positive mindset are usually far better off than those who don't. Not only are they healthier, but they are also more in control of their emotions, have stronger, more satisfying relationships, are often more financially stable and find it easier to achieve goals, pursue ambitions and complete tasks they set themselves. They enjoy deeper sleep, recover quicker from cardiovascular stress and have fewer colds. They don't get as overwhelmed or easily frustrated with the little things in life, which makes them better at dealing with conflict, managing stress and overcoming adversity. There's no point in beating around the bush, the truth is people with a positive mindset are generally happier overall. They also have an easier time dealing with failure and setbacks, often simply seeing them as an opportunity or learning experience from which to grow. On the other hand, people who are negative are habitually deterred further by such circumstances, seeing them as just another example life being unfair and how everything always seems to go wrong.

The good news is that just like everything else, your mindset can be changed, developed and improved with practice. But in order to do so, it's vital you recognise and become aware of the impact caused by your thoughts and emotions, on top of how they influence everything from your health to your behaviour, outlook, relationships and wellbeing. By being aware of the effect they have, you will be able to understand why you reacted to a certain experience the way you did, what you were thinking, and how you were feeling. From there you will be able to adjust your emotional responses and thoughts accordingly, in time being able to recognise and adapt to them as you get them under control.

With that in mind, you shouldn't be trying to be someone else or something you are not, as I genuinely believe that with some hard work, guidance and the right push, you can become the best version of yourself. The reality is your mindset can often hold you back from becoming the person you want to be, which is why you need to honestly believe you can achieve great health and do amazing things. Sure, that sounds easier said than done, but as you continually progress you will develop that self-belief. This is the first step in the direction of realising you are not destined to forever remain in a slump of negative thoughts and emotions, constantly being dragged down by the challenges thrown your way.

Reading that back, it sounds like such a hippyish, pretentious and self-righteous thing to say, that I almost can't believe I'm the one who wrote it. If I was reading that a few years ago I no doubt would have rolled my eyes, laughed and dismissed it. So I won't be offended if you are thinking that now, imagining I'm one of those annoying and overly enthusiastic cheerleader type women you see on TV, shouting empty encouragements like, 'if you just believe in yourself you can become the person you want to be and achieve such great things!'. I've always hated those people and could never stand that patronising 'you can do it' motivation. To me it always seemed so condescending and fake. But I have come to the realisation that we honestly can completely overhaul the way we think about life, improving not only our outlook, but also who we are as people. By accepting that you need to change, and actively embracing it, you can completely change your life for the better.

I know certain parts of what I have discussed so far in this section may come across as naïve, painting a picture of more positive people in a pretentious light, holding hands dancing round a campfire, after carpooling in their Prius. We have all encountered people who are a beacon of positivity, whose presence is quite frankly more annoying than contagious and we actively go out of our way to avoid them. But don't worry; I'm not saying that's who you need to turn into or how you have to behave. What I am however trying to illustrate is the concept of just how much of an impact your mindset has on your overall wellbeing, and how just like everything else, this is a part of your life you can in fact change.

What you need to remember is that people who are generally more positive don't have a stress-free life, void of any challenges or reoccurring instances that get on their nerves. They have just as many negative events or frustrations happen to them on a daily basis, but the difference is they can manage their reactions to them, not letting circumstances out of their control ruin their mood or mindset. That's not to say it never happens, as sure, life's ups and downs inevitably get the better of everyone. But people who are more positive are able to reduce the overall frequency and impact that these events have.

Developing a positive outlook has two main effects on your overall wellbeing. Firstly, it improves your perspective of the world around you, helping inspire creativity and wonder, while encouraging you to explore new options and try new things. Secondly, it develops an emotional resilience that builds up over time, allowing you to flourish and deal with adversity, helping reduce burn out, anxiety and mental aggravation. By consciously working on changing your mindset, reacting in a positive manner will over time become subconscious and automatic. You just need to recognise if there's a problem, then start taking steps to work on it.

Numerous studies have concluded that health and outlook can be directly influenced by the way people view them. Most notable is research conducted by Dr. Cohen at Carnegie Melion University, who took 343 healthy individuals and exposed them to a cold virus. He found that people who were deemed to have a positive emotional mindset or outlook on life had a greater resistance to the virus. Those classified as negative (due to being depressed, anxious or known to have hostile tendencies), were far more likely to claim they had cold-like symptoms, regardless of whether or not they actually developed a cold. This same tendency was seen in another study at John Hopkins University, where by looking at more than 5000 people over the age of 65, it was discovered that the risk of death within the next five years doubled for those who had a poor perception of their health.

But why is this the case?

After an extensive study of how our mindset can be related to our health and mortality, Dr.Engstrom came to the conclusion that it may be due to the increased strain a negative mindset places on the body, causing mental distress. Therefore, mindset could be a huge influence on the development of disease and the performance of the immune system. His research found that individuals who are positive are more likely to have a healthy diet and be more active, factors that have a huge influence on overall health.

In a different study from Duke University, researchers took 3000 people who had significant heart disease and asked them whether they would classify their health as 'poor, fair, good or very good'. It was found that those who chose 'very good' were 70 percent less likely to die within the next three years when compared to those who classified themselves as 'good'. In addition, they had three times the survival rate of people who viewed their health as being 'poor'!

While these studies aren't suggesting that a positive outlook is the only factor related to whether or not you will develop an illness, what they do suggest is that perception can have a huge influence on how the body develops, treats and reacts to disease. If you think back to what I mentioned earlier about how bodily functions don't work optimally when under strain, these findings heavily support the theory as to why people with a positive outlook towards life and their health are far less susceptible to developing illnesses and far more likely to live long and healthy lives. Sure, there will still be influences out of their control such as genetic factors, accidents or simply bad luck. But nothing in life is a certainty and the entire point of improving your mindset is to not only decrease the risks of becoming sick, but also to improve your general happiness, outlook and enjoyment of the time you do have.

"Most people work hard and spend their health trying to achieve wealth.
Then they retire and spend their wealth trying to get back their health."
- Kevin Gianni

Habits

Whether you realise it or not, a large percentage of the decisions you make on a day-to-day basis are due to the habits you have formed. From your routine in the morning, to the first thing you do when you get in at night, the actions you take are often done without even thinking about them. This is because your brain is programmed to function in a certain way and it affects every aspect of your life. On their own, most individual habits are of little relevance. But when combined, they have a huge impact on everything from your health to your financial security, stress levels, productivity, the way you eat and your overall happiness. Whether it's your everyday work routine, the Friday night take away, how often you exercise, or even something as simple as which shoe you put on first, habits play a role in nearly every decision you make. So it really is no exaggeration to say that your routines are an integral part of who you are.

Your brain forms habits based on the actions you perform regularly. By doing so, choices become predetermined, thought processes are eliminated and stress is reduced, making you feel more comfortable as your actions become streamlined. To put it simply, your brain reduces the amount of energy put into daily tasks by going into 'autopilot' mode. In fact, a study published by a researcher at Duke University found that over 40 percent of the actions you perform everyday are simply down to habits.

Meaning that without even realising it, many of the decisions you make, aren't actually decisions at all. For instance, how many food-related choices do you think you make each day? 5? 10? 20?

You will probably be shocked to find that studies out of Cornell University in New York showed that the average person makes 227 food-related choices everyday, most of which are done on a subconscious level. I know this sounds like an insane amount, but it seems that every hour of the day we are faced with choices related to food that we don't even realise, from peeking into the fridge, to walking past a bakery, or the cookies tempting us in the kitchen at work. This makes poor eating habits even more of an issue, since it means we are regularly making uncontrolled decisions that have a negative impact on our health and increasing the control food has over us.

Many of our habits relating to food can be linked back to our childhood. The environment in which we grew up in was the first influence on the times we ate, what we consumed, portion sizes and how we ate our food. Our relationships with food mirrored those of the adults around us and are often a reflection of the rules they put in place, meaning the attitudes we developed towards food as kids directly influences our behaviour as adults. Remember what I said earlier? The general population tends to have a minimal understanding of proper nutrition, or their behaviours and habits in relation to the way they eat. Because of this, society continually passes down these negative actions and behaviours to generation after generation, which in turn, has contributed to the decline of our health and wellbeing.

For instance, many of us were brought up being told we need to finish everything on our plate. While in theory this action is full of good intentions as it's teaching us not to waste food, in reality, all it achieves is forcing us to overeat, developing the mindset and behaviours of eating out of necessity, rather than making a conscious and educated decision to fuel or nourish our body. The consequence of this is that later on as adults we are unable to recognise when or if we are full. This in turn affects our habits as to whether we eat out of hunger, or simply because there's food around to be eaten or in front of us. Be honest, how many times have you picked up a piece of cake or another plate of finger food because it was free at the networking or social event you attended? Or piled up your plate and repeatedly gone back for more at that all you can eat buffet? We rarely go for seconds or thirds when unlimited food is available just because we are hungry, as we seem to approach these situations with the mindset of wanting to make sure the money we paid is well spent, or that we are not missing out when food is provided for free. In these situations we are choosing quantity over quality, with more food equalling more calories being consumed, and often leading to substantial weight gain over a period of time.

Stop and take a moment to think about the meals you have eaten the last few days, including snacks. Which of them were consumed out of hunger? And which were simply because there was food around tempting you to be eaten? Without realising it, it's easy for an occasional afternoon trip to the vending machine or biscuits with your cup of tea to quickly become a daily occurrence. It becomes a feeling of comfort in your mind, something you look forward to and in many cases, gets you through the day. But one study found that while chocolate does boost your mood, that feeling only lasts for three minutes, leaving you in a continuous cycle of chasing those feel-good emotions. If this happens regularly, that occasional treat can quickly just become another part your daily routine. That's right, another habit.

Another example is parents who tell their kids they need to finish all their vegetables to get dessert. Again, while in theory this is full of good intentions, in reality, it creates a habit and mindset that revolves around a reward mechanism. Getting a treat for eating becomes integrated into the child's mind, which causes overeating, since a sugar hit is mentally associated with an empty plate.

Offering a reward for eating all your vegetables also has the negative connotation of depicting vegetables as food that's not enjoyable and therefore deserves a reward for being eaten. In principle it seems so harmless. Chocolate pudding seems like a fair trade off for the health benefits of finishing their broccoli, but on a deeper level it ingrains a long-term association with how they view and approach meals. This in turn can cause people to subconsciously view vegetables as a product they should dislike, associating it with displeasure, which is the complete opposite of what the parents were aiming for. It's not uncommon for this approach to develop into a behaviour where people don't feel satisfied without an evening dessert, regardless of how much they have eaten. That occasional treat develops into a daily event - again, a habit. Personally, this was a huge barrier I had to overcome when improving how I ate, as for a long period of time after every meal, regardless of what or how much I ate, I always craved sugar.

Another issue with this is your brain subconsciously acts out of impulse. This is very similar to a habit, as it becomes almost like a reflex or a remote response to the environment around you, as your brain becomes trained or has accepted this action as a positive one. As you can see being impulsive doesn't just apply to personality traits such as being naturally aggressive or a shop-a-holic, as it can easily affect our eating habits as well. The problem with impulsive eating is that it leads to a loss of physiological control; as we simply can't stop ourselves from taking another bite or reaching for another chip. To top it off, it is an action that can in some instances be completely mindless. It has been found on countless occasions that when asked to recall their daily calorie intake not only do most people underestimate how many calories they have consumed, but they also regularly completely forget about snacks all together, regardless of how often they have them. It's only when their intake is monitored or tracked that they realise how much they are actually indulging, a realisation that more often than not comes as a huge shock and wakeup call as to how detrimental their behaviour truly is. While you may not think it's a big deal, those daily habits can add up to hundreds, if not thousands of extra calories on a weekly basis. This isn't just a problem related to food though, as you will see in due course that detrimental habits can be formed around all aspects of your daily behaviours and decisions.

To truly progress into a healthier lifestyle you need to honestly evaluate your daily actions and find the associations between decisions made because of your habits, or because of what you actually need. Negative habits aren't just related to food though and can just as easily be linked to other actions affecting your wellbeing as well. For instance, always taking the lift or driving to the shops instead of walking, or constantly checking social media, emails or your phone, leading to procrastination or a mind that's always on the go and unable to switch off.

Improving your health will in many ways be a culmination of small changes that on their own may not seem like much, but when added together have a huge effect. This is essential as it helps to avoid feelings of being overwhelmed, which studies have proven can affect your mindset in such a way that you revert back to your old habits, sometimes even sinking deeper into them than before. This is exactly what makes people who go on heavily restrictive diets snap and go back to their old ways, often causing them to regain more weight than they originally lost. It's also what causes people who hop onto the latest fitness trends to quickly lose all motivation, as they become even more deterred by the thought of increasing activity levels than before.

"Motivation is what gets you started. Habit is what keeps you going"
- Jim Rohn

Developing new habits

Every habit you have now was a conscious decision you made at some point in time, from when you have breakfast, to taking up a new hobby, joining a gym or what time you wake up for work. Overtime these actions became automatic and part of your daily routine. This is because your brain is highly responsive to experiences and adaptive to change, which means the good news is you can reprogram the way that it works, as it's able to recognise new experiences and adapt. Through practice, focus and consistency, you will train your mind to break bad old habits and replace them with new ones. This is the true secret behind controlling your weight and developing a long-term, sustainable, healthy lifestyle. The best part about creating new habits is that once they are developed, they become automatic and you no longer even have to think about, work on, or force them. They simply become part of the way your brain functions and subsequently, how you behave.

Having said that, it's important to be mindful that the process often takes work, isn't always easy and does take time. In fact, findings show that depending on how large the change is, new habits can take anything from 21 to 66 days to become a part of your routine. I know that sounds daunting, as the thought alone can be demoralising. Therefore, getting yourself in the right frame of mind before you begin to introduce change is crucial, as you can't let yourself become overwhelmed and unmotivated by the fact that change isn't going to happen overnight. In order to be successful you need to mentally dedicate yourself to creating new habits, and it all starts with understanding why you must replace old ones with better actions that add nourishment and fulfilment to your life. Do you know why you want to do it? Is it your health that's being affected by bad habits? Is it your children's wellbeing? Do you truly want to do it? If you do then you need to accept now that you will need to push yourself during challenging times, as there will be moments when it gets tough and you feel like giving up.

That's why it's all about gradual change, as this helps disruptive actions (such as forced changes in habits) to become less noticeable to our day to day lives. This kind of approach aims to maintain a balance between small lifestyle compromises and what you would habitually be doing otherwise. The problem is that with factors such as work, family commitments or outside influences, is so many people are completely overwhelmed that they can't even contemplate change. In fact, it's not even something they have time to think about, let alone being on the priority list. For that reason, we need to change your mindset in a way that you consciously focus on pursuing healthier actions, regardless of the perceived belief that you don't have the time or that they may be inconvenient.

While these changes may seem unnerving, always remember that in time, they will become second nature, and the habits you develop will be improving your life, not damaging it, meaning that in the times you do choose to indulge, you will be able to enjoy it so much more.

"We become what we repeatedly do."

- Sean Covey

Activity 2

Where to start

Creating new habits is the foundation on which this book and your new lifestyle is based, and because of that I wanted to lay the groundwork for your journey to becoming the best version of yourself.

As a starting point, to get you used to practicing new habits and implementing healthy actions, there are three habit-based changes I want you to add to your daily routine. These can easily be done, regardless of how busy you are. The aim is to ensure you achieve them each and every day, as remember the only way new habits are formed is through continual and repeated use. The entire purpose of this activity is to get you used to making changes so that you establish a solid foundation to build on as you progress. Yes, this will take some focus, commitment and effort, but I selected these changes as they aren't overwhelming, in addition to being relatively easy to act upon and track every day, with the added bonus of having a huge impact on your health.

Habit 1: Add a portion of vegetables or fruit to every meal

By now you are no doubt sick of hearing how you should be eating five portions of fruit and vegetables each day, but from a health perspective, I genuinely can't stress enough how important this truly is. Your body needs a range of vitamins and minerals to perform everyday tasks, from growth to repair or fighting off disease. Failing to consume adequate amounts of these food groups can lead to a whole host of health problems and can be directly linked to many of the issues discussed thus far. It's because of this that before trying to change anything else in your diet, you should first aim to increase your intake, with at least two of these portions coming from a green leafy variety, such as broccoli or spinach, due to the health boosting properties and nutrients they provide.

If you are currently consuming less than your five a day, then I want you to focus on ensuring you add at least one portion to each meal. How and what you include is however entirely up to you. I know five portions may sound like a lot, but if you look at it properly, it's not difficult to find a way to fit them in. For instance, you could add a piece of fruit with breakfast or as a snack, include some spinach in your lunch and a couple of servings of other vegetables to dinner and you are there.

Habit 2: Find ways to walk more on a daily basis

Walking is a great place to start when trying to become more active and it's something everyone should be aiming to do more of, regardless of their current fitness level. Government recommendations state you should aim to walk around 10,000 steps a day, but initially I want you to get yourself into the habit of actively finding ways to walk at least 30 minutes a day. While at first glance on paper that sounds like it will take up a large chunk of your day, it's important to remember that it doesn't need to be done continuously, meaning that you can easily break it up throughout the day and fit it in wherever works best for you.

It may not seem like it, but regardless of how busy you are there are always ways to add more walking into your day-to-day schedule. For instance, walking to get lunch, taking a ten minute walk around the block before meals, having a five minute walking break every couple of hours to stretch your legs, walking to the shops, or even parking in the furthest space away. Yes, I know it may sound like hassle or inconvenience, but the entire point is to start getting into the mindset of finding ways to move more. This will improve your cardiovascular system, which in turn will help you have an easier time with adapting or getting used to any future activities.

There are even a whole host of apps you can use to track your steps so you can see your daily average and how you are progressing.

Habit 3: Drink more water

Your body is made up of around 60 percent water, so it's no surprise that it's required for the majority of everyday functions and that insufficient intake can have a huge impact on your health. In fact, while you can survive for up to a month without food, you would only last a week without water. Most people don't consume anywhere near enough of it and dehydration can be linked to a whole host of negative side effects, including: headaches, exhaustion, dizziness, irritability, low energy and even nausea. It's also common place for people to confuse feelings of thirst with hunger, which can lead to unnecessary snacking or overeating, and can be directly linked to continual weight gain. It's essential you aim to drink at least two to three litres a day, with the amount required varying from person to person depending on their body composition, activity levels and even location. Because of that, I want you to focus on ensuring you increase your intake as much as you can, with the goal being a minimum of two litres.

Personally, I have found the easiest way to keep track of your water intake is to fill a water bottle in the morning, keep it with you at all times and ensure it's finished by the end of the day. Another good habit to introduce is starting your day by drinking one or two glasses first thing in the morning when you get up. Not only will this help you wake up, but it will also kick start your body's functions, as it becomes dehydrated during the night. If you are aiming to lose weight, try having a glass of water around 15 minutes before meals, as this will help cut down on overeating. You can even do the same thing when you are tempted to snack, as that's the best way to determine whether you are actually hungry, or merely just thirsty. Chances are, this will help the cravings to pass.

If you are prone to fizzy drinks or hot beverages, start small by swapping out every other drink. If plain water is not your thing, then make it more interesting by drinking flavoured water or green teas, add some lemon, lime, orange or cucumber slices, or even some ginger, mint or a variety of other herbs and flavourings. Whatever you do though, try to avoid cordials or anything with high amounts of sugar, artificial sweeteners or any other empty calories.

Summary

From now on, each and every day I want you to:

1) Add a portion of vegetables or fruit to every meal
2) Aim to walk at least 30 minutes a day
3) Ensure you up your water intake

"Much of the stress that people feel doesn't come from having too much to do. It comes from not finishing what they've started."
- David Allen

The importance of having a goal

In the introduction I mentioned how my past mindset put a huge toll on my health. I used to be full of negative emotions, failing to see the good in life, easily overwhelmed and feeling like I was stuck in a never-ending rut. Being rarely happy and unable to see the good in things put a huge strain on my health, relationships and wellbeing. I doubt I was much fun to be around, always moping and finding something to complain about. But what I learned in the last few years is that often what it takes to break away from this state of mind is to become inspired, as developing a purpose in life can completely change the way you look at things. Unfortunately, you can't force inspiration, but what I have found, is that becoming goal orientated and having something to work towards is often the easiest way to inspire yourself from within, and change your outlook.

When dealing with new clients, I find one reoccurring theme that not only negatively affects their lifestyle, but also has a huge impact on their ability to adapt to and embrace change: their lack of having a clear goal.

You will always come across people who complain endlessly about life, the hand they have been dealt or circumstances they are in. Yet they never actively try to change their situation. Someone I used to work with comes to mind as the perfect example of this, as he would spend all day whining about how much he hated his job. He would turn up looking miserable and progressively worsen throughout the day, acting like a more realistic version of grumpy, without the other six dwarves. In his mind everything that was wrong in his life was always someone or something else's fault, but no matter how much he complained, he would never actually try and do anything about it. Regardless of how bad things were, he never took it upon himself to own up to his responsibility for his circumstances and at the time of writing he was still sat in the same position after nine years. In fact, he was one of the big motivators that made me realise that was a life I didn't want to have anymore and it forced me to push myself to chase more. A life like that isn't living, it's merely existing and I couldn't think of anything worse than nearly a decade later being sat in exactly the same situation feeling sorry for myself. But the unfortunate reality is it's far easier to sit back, moan and accept how things are, than to actively make changes, which is why so many people get stuck where they are. In a way, this can be put down to change often being perceived or associated with risk, which for many people is an uncomfortable feeling they would rather avoid. We have probably all fallen into this state at one time or another, as it's human nature to want to be comfortable and not face adversity, which is why it's so important to keep pushing yourself if you want to continue to grow. If you don't, then before you know it you will be reaching retirement, having spent the last 30 years in a job or environment you hate, full of habits that are negatively impacting your health and regretting having wasted what little time you have left.

Part of the process of developing a more positive mindset is recognising and accepting that things can't be good all of the time and it's unavoidable that on occasion challenges will arise that push you, your patience and your nerves. However, it's the way you deal with setbacks during these moments that define your overall state of mind. Losing yourself in issues that you drag with you for days and days, in the back of your mind and adding them to the negative pile will only kill your psychological wellbeing, placing a never ending strain on your health. Which unfortunately for many people is a reality from which they never escape.

This is why I want to stress the importance of goal setting, as without it I would most likely still be stuck in that situation. I found that simply having something to work towards and making small steps in progressing towards it every day, drastically changed my outlook on life.

The misperception of failure

It's an undeniable truth that nobody likes to fail, and for most of us the fear of failure is what prevents us from pursuing what we really want in life on a personal, professional and emotional level. Instead of putting ourselves out there, we would rather do whatever we can to avoid the negative feelings that come with failing. But what we don't realise is that as hard as it may seem, it's often from failure that we learn the most; we learn who we are, what we're capable of, our strengths, weaknesses and how to keep from repeating the same mistakes in the future.

In many cases failure can even lead you down a different path than you otherwise would have found yourself on, which is why you shouldn't be scared of failing. Instead, you should be scared of never pushing yourself to find out what you are truly capable of. This is why you need to learn to view failure as an opportunity for personal growth and development. Thomas Edison put it best when he said; 'I have not failed, I have simply found 10,000 ways that will not work'. But without trying, you will never find the way that will.

A big part of changing and improving any aspect of your life will come down to pushing your comfort zones. While I understand that this is probably an extremely scary prospect, the way you need to look at it is that your comfort zones will continue to expand as you try new things. Because of that every step you take outside those zones, no matter how small, causes them to expand, making that your new comfort zone. That's why I'm such a proponent of taking small gradual steps, as they make you more comfortable at trying new things, inevitably raising your confidence in all areas of life.

"The difference between the impossible and the possible lies in a person's determination."

- Tommy Lasorda

Continual goal setting

It's important that you set yourself new goals, not just in weight loss, fitness, or your time during this process, but in your continued development of becoming a better you. In many ways, having a goal provides what many people are lacking: a purpose or reason to get up in the morning. They keep you going when times get tough and act as a reminder about why you started in the first place. Not only that, but they also give you something to mentally focus on and strive towards. Then, when you do make time to relax and unwind, you can do so knowing you have earned and deserve it, which provides a sense of mental peace and balance, relieving feelings of guilt or self-doubt. Setting goals for yourself doesn't have to be an intimidating prospect either, but with that in mind it's important to make sure they are both realistic and achievable.

When I was younger I learned this lesson the hard way, as I set my mind on the goal of becoming a 'rock star' at the expense of everything else. Was it achievable and realistic? No. But it did teach me a lot about what I did want to do and how to get there, all the while keeping me sane by giving me something to aspire to be. I spent my younger years completely fixated on this idea and in hindsight it was because I had absolutely no clue what else I wanted to do. So I latched onto the one thing that could help me possibly avoid the reality of what I definitely knew I didn't want, which was a dead end nine to five office job, where I'd spend my days aimless wasting away starring at a clock. Which as you read earlier, is exactly where I ended up.

So when I talk about failure and growing from it, my experience is a prime example. No, I'm not headlining in music arenas around the world, but having goals, ambitions and pushing myself when I was knocked down led me to places I would have never found otherwise. The process helped me discover not only what I'm good at, but also what I enjoy, leading me down a path where I can apply my passion for writing and helping people to a field that ten years ago I never would have dreamed I'd be in.

It's amazing how much our views and perceptions of the world, who we are and what we enjoy can change as we become exposed to new situations and experiences. Ten years ago I couldn't have imagined anything worse than thinking about what I ate or getting up early to go to the gym, which is why I completely understand and empathise with people over how difficult change can be. Yet now, these are both aspects that are a part of my life that I not only enjoy, but also look forward to and get huge satisfaction out of. In the end all that really matters is that what you do makes you happy and gives you a sense of fulfilment, as both of these are vital to achieving mental clarity and improving your mindset.

Goals don't have to be big for them to be life changing either, and often short-term goals can make a process easier, since the journey can be broken down into smaller, more achievable steps. This could mean simply finding ways to free up 30 minutes for yourself in the evening a couple of nights a week to relax, or you could choose to incorporate regular activities in your evening such as going for a run, spending more time with your loved ones, or ensuring every meal has at least one serving of vegetables.

When I talk about having a goal, it means you need to have a plan, a path, a direction and an action, not just a misguided short-term target looking for a quick fix. A large part of your personal growth will be based on becoming accountable to yourself for your own actions, therefore having a goal forces you to put together a plan of how to achieve it. This is essential in all parts of your life, as things don't happen if you don't put them down, attach a date, do research, determine how much it will cost and decide how to get there. It is only by doing so that a thought becomes real, and the more specific you are, the easier it becomes to both recognise and resolve problems. Not having a plan means you have a lack of control, which is why the more you can see, touch and feel, the less stress will come with it.

Chances are, that structure is exactly what has been missing for you in the past and why you have struggled to progress, as all the good intentions in the world can't stop you from drifting off course when you haven't got something to help you stick to it, which is why the biggest hurdle to getting started is often taking the first step. In one way or another everyone is guilty of putting things off and delaying what needs to be done, and the worst part is, this occurs even more so with things you are not held accountable for, which are often the things you need to do most. Unfortunately, this is true regardless of how much, deep down, you believe you want it. Simply wanting to do something, in and of itself, is not enough of a motivator to get it accomplished. After all, how many times have you missed the gym because you were too tired? Put off studying till tomorrow? Ordered a take away because you didn't feel like cooking?

It's easy to say that from tomorrow 'I'm going to go to the gym three times a week' or 'I'm going to spend 30 minutes a day working on my French'. Without a plan or schedule though, there isn't much apart from your willpower or mood the next day that can stop you from procrastinating about it again. Combine this with life's everyday stresses which happen more often than not, and you can easily see why unstructured goals fall by the wayside. Setting deadlines for when you want to achieve certain parts of your goals helps instil not only a feeling of accountability, but also a progressive mindset that it's actually happening, you can see results and you are the one driving them! Starting and stopping and getting round to it whenever you are in the mood will yield little to no progress, instead all it will do is keep your goal in the back of your mind and in time will likely make it become something you always wanted to do, but forgot about or never got around to, making it just another dream or desire to add to your list of regrets or 'what ifs'.

I'm sure everyone has lay in in bed late at night thinking about what they want to achieve, the changes they want to make and what they need to do to sort their lives out. In the moment full of motivation, thinking that tomorrow will be a new day and a fresh start, where everything finally comes together. But how many people can honestly say they woke up the next morning and got on with the changes? I know there have been countless times I haven't, as that restless night's sleep just leaves you feeling drained, having lose any desire you may have conjured.

Instead the easier option is always to put it off and just accept the way things are, which tends to be the route so many of us take. My dad always told me 'the easiest option is rarely the right one' and I think that holds true with most things in life. Therefore, by making a plan with a timeline that's incorporated into your life as an essential part of your day, makes it far easier to find the motivation to go through with what you want to accomplish. Getting started is always the hard part, but as with most things, once you get into a routine and develop a habit it becomes far easier.

It's important on your continued journey of self-improvement to find new things you want to achieve, as this will allow you to set new goals and continue to push yourself throughout your life. But on the other side of that, it's also important to find a balance. So whatever you aim to do, do it for the right reasons, as it's far easier to get something done if you are passionate about it, or at least have an interest in doing it. Without that drive you will struggle to find the motivation to stick with it, which is why it's essential to make sure the goals you set are realistic. Far too many people read about fad diets and crazy work outs online, make radical changes in their lives only to give up shortly thereafter. The goal and end result they built up in their mind simply wasn't achievable within the timeframe they desired and most importantly, it wasn't something they enjoyed either. Thereby meaning even if they did progress, it wouldn't be maintainable long-term. I have met and spoken to so many people who dive straight into the latest fitness plans, map out a whole new diet and radically overhaul their lives. Completely focused and committed to the idea that this time they are finally going to do it and change their lives. Then, a few days in, they get in one night too tired to work out. They don't feel like cooking and they tell themselves it's ok, they will just take this one night off, as surely they have earned it after being good for a few days. Then the same thing happens the next night and the next. By the following week the entire notion is completely dismissed and replaced by excuses as to why it wasn't for them, that they don't have the time, or are just not someone who can do something like that.

Visualisation will be a hugely powerful tool for keeping you motivated and on track, even during the toughest of times. Not just in regards to developing a healthier lifestyle, but also because you will be able to apply the techniques you are learning to all aspects of your life. It will help you keep pushing forward, even when you feel like giving up.

Even if this entire concept still seems like a daunting prospect to you, trust me when I say that once you start achieving goals and realising more of what you are capable of, it will be a natural reaction to try and see what you can do next. Achieving goals will boost your confidence, as you strive to find your true potential. I know this all still sounds a bit too feel good and positive, but achieving something you previously thought was impossible will give you a renewed sense of vigour, making you question what other challenges you can overcome if you simply put your mind to it.

For those of you feeling trapped and overwhelmed, don't worry you are not alone. As you have seen so far I've been there myself many times in my life, which is why I have tried to share some personal stories about what I have been through and how I've dealt with it. With that in mind I'd like to take a moment to tell you about how I got to the point I'm at now, my journey getting here and how I finally got out of the mindset of feeling completely helpless and lost.

My greatest revelation

When first meeting me, most people would in all likelihood jump to the conclusion that since I write about and work in health, nutrition and fitness that it has always been an interest and passion of mine. But as I have already expressed, that couldn't be further from the truth. Growing up I was never into sports, sure, I tried on rare occasions, but I was never athletically gifted and to put it quite bluntly, I sucked at pretty much everything I tried. From football to volleyball or rugby, you name it, if it involved coordination or sudden movements, then there was a 99 percent chance I'd be rubbish at it. On top of that, while I was never obese, I was always the guy who was a bit chubby and overweight. I was never happy with myself or my body, which led to low levels of confidence, self-doubt and insecurities to the point where most of the time I was too embarrassed to take my shirt off at the beach. I couldn't think of anything I wanted to do less than enter a gym or worry about what I ate and the entire concept of personal wellbeing was so foreign to me, that it never even crossed my mind. I regularly lived off fast food and spent a large amount of my time in bars or indoors playing video games.

Even in my early twenties I had already pretty much given up and accepted that this was how my life was meant to be and do you know what? Looking back, I was kind of OK with it, as I had never known anything different and that had always been the world I had lived in. Then in my mid-twenties I got talked into going to a local gym with a friend. I didn't really take it seriously, as it was something I got dragged into and didn't overly enjoy or want to do. I mainly turned up, half arsed the workouts and made excuses to myself as to why I couldn't push myself properly. Eventually I moved and stopped training with my friend, but I had got into the habit of going to the gym so stuck with it. My mindset and approach however pretty much stayed the same over the next couple of years, regularly skipping workouts and still paying no attention to my diet. To this day I still remember the moment everything changed and I decided to turn it all around. I was on a beach on holiday, surrounded by well-built guys who all had six packs and I decided I was tired of feeling inferior or self-conscious about how I looked. So I set myself a goal of hitting 10 percent body fat by the following summer and started working towards it.

Did I do it? No, I didn't even come close as it was far too unrealistic. Especially since I had no clue what I was doing, let alone any idea of how the body worked, the type of training I should be focusing on, or how I should be eating. I also still bought heavily into much of the misleading information you find in the latest trends. Even though my progress was limited, the important thing was that I had a goal, something I was working towards, and a reason to get myself to exercise, even when I didn't want to.

This is probably not the feel good 'look how amazing I am and what I did' story you were expecting. But the reason I am sharing it is that what the continual grind eventually did for me was spark an interest in my own wellbeing. That interest combined with the shock of my dad's cancer diagnosis and the fear of having that happen to me led me to decide that not only did I need to get healthy, but that if I was going to do it, I was going to do it properly. So I set about learning as much about health, nutrition and fitness as I possibly could. Sure, I still made a lot of mistakes along the way, but that's just part of the process, and as I already said, often some the greatest lessons are learned through these failures. The experience taught me the right and wrong way to be doing things, where I needed to apply more focus and what aspects needed more work.

It wasn't all positive though. At the time, I was miserable with my life and stuck in a job I hated. But having a goal of what I wanted to achieve helped to keep me going and it at least gave me an outlet that in many ways kept me sane. My unhappiness was largely caused by the company and environment I was in, along with the dreaded nine to five, where, like so many others, I was trapped due to the common issue faced by most people these days: starting from the bottom to get experience. I also I had bills to pay and I do like being able to eat, so for a while I simply accepted my situation and got on with it, as the way I saw it there wasn't a better alternative and it needed to be done.

About a year down the line I finally got an opportunity that I thought would make everything better. I had an interview at a top marketing agency, for a position filled with all the fancy clients, progression, perks and benefits I had convinced myself I needed to be happy. It was the chance that would make all the long days and what felt like endless suffering I put myself through worthwhile. Mid-interview though I had a moment of self-realisation. I realised it wasn't my job I hated, it was my entire career. While discussing what would be involved with the new role it dawned on me that it simply sounded terrible, and something I would get no enjoyment or fulfilment out of. It was just a path I had fallen into because I had no idea what I wanted to do, so I had forced myself into a situation where I was adhering to societal norms and what was expected of me. But I knew right there and then that I needed a change or I would never be happy and somehow in that moment I realised what my true passion was. I went home that night and laid out a plan based on what I wanted to do. I cancelled my move to a new city and registered to be a student again, as I decided I wanted to study nutrition.

Sure, this change was terrifying. It meant taking a huge risk and staying stuck in an unhappy situation for the foreseeable future while I got qualified and set about starting my business. But overnight, my mindset completely changed. I felt a huge relief, like a massive, overwhelming burden had been lifted. I was a long way from where I wanted to be, but by taking control for the first time I could actually visualise a situation in the future in which I would not only be doing something I was passionate about, but I'd also be happy doing it.

Don't get me wrong, everything didn't suddenly become magically better. There continued to be bad days in a draining and challenging environment. I was still struggling mentally and emotionally. But now my mindset was stronger than ever and I truly believed that in the long run it would all be worthwhile. My goal of wanting to write a book and start a health coaching company meant a lot of late nights and early mornings, hard work and sacrifices. But the visualisation of what I wanted and where I wanted to be kept me going, and it continually pushed me to strive to be better. I embraced and enjoyed the journey and found out I could do and achieve things I never thought possible. The closer I got to achieving my goal, the more my mindset improved. It completely changed my outlook on life and brought out the best possible version of who I am, a version of myself I never thought I could be, and someone I would like if I met him.

What was the point of this story?

Hopefully that story gives you an idea of how drastically life can change and why I stand by what I am teaching you, as I have been right there in the trenches going through it myself. This is why I stress the importance of continual goal setting, as a mere goal of getting healthier opened my eyes to what I was truly passionate about, in a field I had absolutely no interest in while I was growing up.

The big takeaway point is that if I hadn't of set targets and tried to push myself, I would never have discovered my interest in health or nutrition, and I would most likely still be stuck being miserable, staring at a clock all day as life passed me by. Sure, you could argue I got lucky and fell into what I wanted to do, but it would never have happened if I hadn't forced myself to push my comfort zones and make a change in the first place. The entire point of this section was to inspire you to find new ways to challenge yourself, move out of your comfort zone and experience new things. By doing this and exposing yourself to new experiences, you give yourself the opportunity to discover what you truly enjoy and what you actually want in life.

The aim of this section was to get you motivated to want to set goals and start your journey, but it is important to remember that your enthusiasm can work against you if you aren't careful. It's easy to throw yourself head first into a new and exciting venture, full of ambition and drive, ready to give it your all. But the reality is there is such a thing as working too much for your goal, to the point where you actually work against it. Going from one extreme to another can quickly cause you to burn yourself out and believe me when I say I'm talking from experience on this one, as I learned the lesson that you can be too driven and push things too far.

When I first started out writing this book and setting up my business, I was working ridiculously long hours, as I knew the sooner I could get it done, the sooner I could change my situation. At first it wasn't an issue, but after a while the 16 hour days were no longer sustainable. My work started to suffer and as I said earlier, this caused my cortisol and stress levels to shoot through the roof. I was mentally, physically, and emotionally drained, and the lack of balance tipped the scale further in the direction of negatively impacting my health.

No matter how much you want it or how hard you are willing to work, it's essential you enforce some form of balance between working towards your goals and actually having a life. If you don't, what's the point of it all if you don't have a good life? By all means work hard and chase your dreams, but take time to enjoy the little things in life as well. Break a sweat, see the world, enjoy good food and dance the night away. Appreciate the company you have, the opportunities you receive and ensure you properly rest, relax and recover. Most importantly though, embrace everything that life has to offer, make the most of the journey and don't just fixate on the end result, as before you know it time will have passed you by. So make all the memories and stories that cement your legacy along the way.

"Without reflection, we go blindly on our way, creating more unintended consequences, and failing to achieve anything useful."
- **Margaret J. Wheatley**

Activity 3

Self reflection

Before moving on I'd like you to spend some time reflecting on your life, taking into account what you have learned from the content covered so far and what it has made you realise about yourself.

I want you to think about:

1) What does being fit and healthy mean to you?
2) What parts of your life do you want to change?
3) What do you want to achieve?

You can make these notes on the 'Mindset' activity sheet in the downloadable content pack over at:
www.tailoredlifestyles.co.uk/activities

What you come up with will be one of the focus points in the final section, so I highly recommend that you take some time and really think about your answers before carrying on. Like I said before, this is one of the activities that in the long run, the more you put into it, the more you will get out of the process.

Your answers could be anything from having the energy to play with your kids, no longer getting out of breath when you walk, eating healthier, or finding time for yourself to relax. Or maybe you want to spend 15 minutes a day reading a book, finally start that course to further develop your career, or build up to running a half marathon. There are no right or wrong answers and I want you to put down whatever is important to you. It doesn't matter how many ideas you come up with either. If anything, the more the merrier, as that will give you more to work with at a later date, as we tailor your journey around you.

Give this some proper thought before moving on.

Pillar Two
Exercise

"Physical fitness is not only one of the most important keys to a healthy body, it is the basis of dynamic and creative intellectual activity."
- John F. Kennedy

It seems that everywhere you look these days you are told you need to find ways to be more active, with suggestions ranging from joining a gym to attending a class, taking the stairs or even walking instead of driving whenever you can. Yet research shows roughly 80 percent of people in the UK and USA don't reach the recommended levels of 30 minutes of activity five times a week, which is a clear sign that something drastically needs to be done. Even more shocking were the findings in one of the most comprehensive studies ever conducted in the UK. The research found that with the exception of when they went food shopping, one in ten people hadn't even walked continually for more than five minutes during the four week time frame in which they were questioned!

In a world of continually evolving technology and with jobs becoming increasingly more sedentary, it seems inactivity has simply become a part of people's lives. The problem is that these days it's far too easy to avoid having to move or do anything you don't want to do and it doesn't take an expert to see how this all relates to the issues we saw earlier in this book. Things don't seem to be getting any better either, as people are becoming increasingly reliant, expectant and dependant on convenience.

Addiction to television and social media combined with high stress and sedentary jobs has created a generation of overwhelmed couch potatoes, going from one seated position staring at a screen all day to another all night, with little reason or incentive to move. Apart from their health that is, but moving and being more active is something very few people seem to be considering. This is made even worse in a world where businesses are making substantial profits by finding ways in which to minimise processes and offer services that require as little effort as possible from the consumer. If drive thru fast food restaurants where you don't even have to get out your car weren't bad enough, it's now got to the point where you can place orders at the touch of a button and get lunch delivered straight to your desk at work. Meaning many people fail to engage in any physical activity or even take a few hundred steps a day, let alone the 10,000 steps recommended by governmental guidelines. On the surface it may not seem consequential, but over time, all those instances when you turn to convenience in order to avoid any effort add up, and they have a substantial influence on not only on how you feel, but also on your ingrained habits, decisions, behaviours and long-term health.

But do you know what, I get it. I get that when you are busy the last thing you want to worry about is 'wasting' time walking to get lunch. I get that after a long day even taking the stairs feels exhausting, let alone thinking about finding the energy to go for a run or to the gym. I get that it's far easier to just have a routine of getting home exhausted and not wanting to move from the sofa. After all, who am I to judge? I used to be exactly like that. I wouldn't walk or move anywhere I didn't have to and I couldn't bear the thought of building up a sweat or entering a gym. And you could forget the idea of going outside and getting some fresh air, as who knows, it could be cold out there, it might rain, or I might have to engage directly with people rather than from behind a computer screen. And there's always the risk of missing an important moment in the rerun of a show I'd already seen.

These examples of reasons to avoid exercise may seem pathetic or exaggerated, but as bad as they sound, it's excuses and justifications like these that far too many people make (mostly to themselves) each and every day. I even used to joke that I learned to drive so I wouldn't have to walk anywhere I didn't have to, and do you know what? Deep down, part of me actually meant it. There was always a reason or excuse that validated for me why I didn't need to do something. Eventually though, without even thinking about it, I always resorted to the easiest option, as that's exactly what avoiding moving, being active or doing exercise is: the easy option. The sad reality is that mindset made me just like the majority of people, who neglect this part of their health.

The problem is modern society has adapted to having no real need to move. Everything seems to have an easier alternative and we have gotten used to and like being comfortable, not having to push ourselves or leave our comfort zones. Because of that we have developed an outlook where the hassle of having to exert ourselves far outweighs the perceived risks of not doing so. Don't get me wrong, I completely understand the lack of desire, energy or motivation to force yourself into engaging in an activity you don't think you'd enjoy, especially when it means adding yet another item to that never ending list of things to do. With how stressful and overwhelming people's lives have become, it's no surprise that this aspect of their health always seems to be relegated to the bottom of the list of priorities until it is too late.

But with that being said, the lack of motivation to be active can't be blamed on ignorance. Everyone knows they should be doing more and it's safe to say that the majority of people are well aware of the risks involved. It has even reached the point where advances in medical science along with the acceptance of radical procedures has made reducing the size of your stomach surgically, or having your fat sucked out, more appealing than tackling ingrained habits and getting directly to the root of the problem.

"Those who think they have no time for exercise will sooner or later have to find time for illness."

- Edward Stanley

But does it really matter?
Is exercise really that important for our health?

As you can probably guess, the short answer to that question is, yes it is. Studies have undeniably confirmed the health benefits of being more active. In fact, the American Heart Association even goes as far as claiming that for every hour you exercise, you add two hours to your life. But if that isn't enough of an incentive, then there are an array of other benefits too, from reducing the risk of cardiovascular disease by improving blood cholesterol levels to controlling, normalising or even preventing high blood pressure. A few other benefits include reducing stress, improving flexibility, helping avoid osteoporosis by developing stronger bones and muscles, boosting your mood and giving you more energy. Not only that, exercise has been found to make you more confident. Not just in how you look and feel, but also through the achievement of goals and targets. Pushing yourself and realising what you are capable of gives you increased feelings of self-worth and a belief in yourself, making you more productive and more likely to try and take on new challenges. Furthermore, the risk of developing certain cancers such as lung, colon and breast are lowered, arthritis pain can be eased and overall quality of life is dramatically improved. Basically, the majority of health issues our modern world is currently facing on mental, physical and emotional levels could be treated, improved or even resolved, simply by finding ways to move more on a daily basis.

Earlier, we explored the problems caused by having a negative mindset, with problems including but not limited to, depression, anxiety, stress and anger issues. Studies have proven exercise to be one of the best tools to positively influence and counteract these outlooks, because it affects you on both a physiological and psychological level.

In fact, regular exercise has been proven to be one of, if not the most effective treatment for some forms of depression, with studies showing an increase in activity is as good, if not better than the pills prescribed for mild to moderate cases. It also has the added benefit of not having any side effects or negative reactions to the toxins pills place on the body on a daily basis. Research suggests that exercise's success in the treatment of depression can be linked to giving participants a feeling of self-worth and positive self-regard. By successfully proving to the individual that they can change the type of person they believe they are and become better, it thereby acts as the catalyst or driving force they need to change other aspects of their lives. This can often help people get out of a rut, or act as a push to start the shift in mindset needed to do so. This change in thinking can help them start to believe they are more capable than they originally gave themselves credit for, which aids in alleviating self-doubt and negative thoughts that may have previously caused them to feel trapped or inferior.

On top of that, incorporating exercise into your new healthy lifestyle can help in other areas as well. For instance, it can clear your mind resulting in improved sleep, help you relax, or even give you an outlet to release tensions caused by feelings of pressure or being overwhelmed. For many people a good workout is exactly what they need after a long stressful day to make themselves feel better, as exercise allows them to release all the negative energy and emotions they have built up throughout the day. This links directly to what was discussed previously in regards to the problems brought about by stress and elevated cortisol levels, as exercise has the ability to play a huge role in lowering and controlling both. This is because engaging in physical activity causes your body to release feel good hormones such as dopamine, which metabolises stress hormones and is the reason why you always find you have an improved mood and clearer mindset after working out.

Being more active also aids in stabilising appetite, with research showcasing that poor appetite control is often present in people who are largely sedentary. In turn this is potentially making a massive contribution to overeating and weight gain. Often we turn to food during times of despair and use it as a coping mechanism for relief. The biggest problem with this is that sugar is often the focal point of what we choose to consume. Yet this relief is only temporary, and often simply spurs on further negative feelings and emotions. Therefore, increased activity offers an alternative outlet to turn to during those times. Increasing your physical activity aids in blood sugar management and weight control, which has the knock on effect of lowering the risk of developing chronic diseases and obesity. Exercise also makes participants far more likely to change their eating habits and make healthier food choices. This is because they begin to consciously want to fuel their bodies with the nutrients required to boost performance and help with recovery, as their progress spurs them to want further improve the results they are seeing.

But with all that being said, the honest truth is that out of all four of the areas this book focuses on improving, becoming more active will for many people be the hardest to implement and stick to. This is because for many this concept is by far the most foreign to them and it also requires the most effort both mentally and physically. The statistics simply don't lie, and with the way our world has evolved it seems that people are spending their entire lives fearing or avoiding being active, at all costs. What makes matters even worse is that apathy is now the norm within society, rather than being an exception. This makes it even harder to break away from the temptations and pressure faced everyday. From that extra hour in bed, driving instead of walking to the shops, or skipping class to catch up with the latest shows, there will always be temptations trying to lead you astray, regardless of how motivated or committed you may be.

No matter how difficult it is to eat healthier, find ways to manage stress or relax, in comparison, these will usually be far easier to change than addressing the concept of increasing your physical activity. Finding the motivation to lace up those shoes and get out of the house after a long day, working up the courage to sign up for a class or ask for help will not be easy and it's always harder not to give in to temptations in the initial stages of change. But that doesn't mean it's impossible, as I'm living proof that's far from the case. I'm simply just trying to prepare you for what will no doubt be the most challenging adaptation to becoming a better you.

So while I could keep going on about the positives of increased activity levels for the rest of this chapter, crossing my fingers hoping that something will magically click into place and your mindset will change. I'm unfortunately completely aware that in all likelihood, doing so would have little to no effect, and if anything, might even just be a waste of our time. At the end of the day, I'm not here to preach and the last thing I want to do is to deter you further, as making you feel bad about yourself when you can't understand why you are unable to find the motivation to make an important change like this achieves nothing. This is exactly why I'm so against those 'phoney' you can do it motivational programmes, as many of them lead users into believing that if they can't do it or stick to every word they say then there's something wrong with them. But the reality is regardless of what I could say about the benefits of becoming more active, some of you will still no doubt be thinking that while that's all well and good, you just don't have the time. And even though it may sound like a great idea now, it will be a completely different story as soon as that early morning alarm goes off. The case may even be that as much as you'd like to, you have other desires or commitments you have to prioritise. Or it might simply sound like a lot of hassle, or like it's not something you would want to do or enjoy, regardless of the benefits of doing so.

I know this all may sound overly negative and the last thing you would expect to read in a book about healthy lifestyles, as books like this are traditionally all upbeat and positive. But I promised from the very start I'd be honest and wouldn't beat around the bush in regards to what developing a healthier wellbeing entails. It's undeniably true that the usual upbeat, "you can do it" approach just doesn't work, because everyone knows they should be doing more. In fact, they are constantly told so on a weekly, if not daily basis, yet despite all that, the majority of people simply ignore these warnings. I'm basing this judgement not only on the mindset's of people I have worked with, but also research found in behavioural studies that look at society as a whole. I'm also taking into consideration who I used to be and the way I used to think, as a few years ago my reaction to this information would have been exactly along those lines.

Note how I said 'used to'. Over time I managed to change my way of thinking and found ways to shift priorities and commitments so I could fit being more active into my way of life. In time it actually became something I enjoyed, rather than feared or dismissed. But just because I said there's little use in continuing with this method doesn't mean I'm giving up on the issue. Plus, having this knowledge helps in giving you a little nudge when times get hard, and just like anything else, it doesn't hurt to expand your understanding of how everything covered will improve your overall wellbeing.

So with all that in mind, let's try a different approach. Let's try and get to the bottom of why your current lifestyle is in all likelihood lacking in activity. Let's explore the misconceptions you potentially have that put you off the entire notion of being more active. Let's try to determine what's acting as a deterrent preventing you from embracing this part of your health and let's look at what activities and strategies are available that can help you avoid any hurdles that may arise along the way. When all is said and done this entire book is based around your own tailored journey of self-realisation, and it's about you deciding to do something because it's important to you and you want to do it, not because I told you to. Hopefully by approaching it in this manner you can finally find the desire to change and I'll do my part in providing you with all the knowledge of exactly how to do so. As hard as it may seem, there are and will be ways you can implement exercise into your day-to-day routine, no matter how busy you are, how many other commitments you have, or any other barriers you perceive as getting in the way. Your journey is all about finding those ways and learning how to make them work for you. But most importantly, your journey is about finding out what you enjoy and what enriches your life.

"If we could give every individual the right amount of nourishment and exercise, not too little and not too much, we would have found the safest way to health."

- Hippocrates

A different approach

I'd like to start this new approach with a simple question:

If exercise is so beneficial to people's wellbeing, why are so few of us doing it?

The issue isn't as simple as the media portrays it to be, often touting the reasons for a lack of activity as it being too hard, people not having the time, or simply putting it down to sheer laziness. Sure, for some this may be the case, but the truth is for others there's often a much deeper underlying factor. The truth is that for many of us the idea of engaging in physical activity is an extremely daunting prospect, especially if it's something we have always feared or never understood. Like many things in life, misconceptions have overcomplicated the issue, which in essence, is actually pretty simple. There's no denying some aspects may take practice or time to get used to, but like most things, the key is to start small, don't overthink it and build your way up.

I remember a while ago I read a story about a cancer patient whose doctor said it was necessary to find ways to incorporate exercise into their daily routine. He genuinely believed this wasn't possible, as he didn't have the energy or strength to visit a gym. Through no fault of his own, what he didn't realise was that simply going for walks around the block or through the nearby park would be massively beneficial to his health. Not only would it get him moving, but it would expose him to fresh air, give him time to enjoy his surroundings and help his overall state of mind. Exercise has been proven to greatly improve the quality of life of cancer patients as well as other people with serious illnesses, and has even been linked to helping with treatment and recovery. In the article, the reporter stated that the patient had dismissed the idea of simply walking, as his preconceptions about what was involved with exercise had led him to believe that these actions wouldn't be sufficient enough to achieve anything.

What can we learn from this story?

It's fair to say this is a widespread misconception and a barrier faced by many people who underestimate the positive effects that can be brought on by small actions. Personally I think simply walking more is an amazing place to start when trying to increase your activity levels, as it places a minimal amount of stress on the body and is an activity that most people can comfortably engage in with complete control, and without getting overwhelmed. While at first glance as an action it may not seem like much, several studies have found 30 minutes of brisk walking a day can reduce the risks of developing cardiovascular disease and diabetes by as much as 30 percent. Brisk walking also lowers blood sugar levels and improves the body's response to insulin, with researchers at the University of Boulder Colorado also suggesting that regular walking can reduce the risk of stroke by 20 to 40 percent. So as you can clearly see, this 'small action' can have a profound impact on your overall health.

Unfortunately, society and the media have built up perceptions of exercise being all about big meat-head guys and thin, anorexic girls posing on Instagram. We are constantly shown the latest work out plans and sold on the idea that if you can still stand or haven't thrown up by the end of the session you haven't worked hard enough. This has led people to believe that it takes gruelling hours of exhaustive workouts every week to be healthy, and anything short of that simply isn't worthwhile.

I'm sure everyone can remember those nightmare PE lessons being shouted at in the cold and rain, all while being forced to do an activity you hated and got no enjoyment out of. It's no wonder people are deterred or frightened by the prospect of exercising if they have only ever had negative experiences. Bad memories like these create a misguided preconception that all activities are the same, when in fact, the likelihood is that there is going to be some form of activity to suit everyone. Even now as someone who regularly works out, when I think back on some of my past experiences with being active, the idea completely puts me off. At school I pretty much dreaded all of the sports and activities we were thrown into and that's part of the reason why I lived a sedentary life for so long. Those experiences tarnished all forms of exercise in my mind and I labelled them all as something I wouldn't enjoy.

This is why I can completely empathise and understand why someone who has never really tried to be active has complete disassociation with the concept. Especially since it's portrayed as primarily for people they can't relate to and don't want to be like. A lot of people whom I have met have been apprehensive about joining a gym, attending a class or taking up an activity, viewing them as only being for 'fit' people and not something they could do. It's human nature to fear or avoid what we don't understand, especially if we feel like we won't fit in, which is why if there's ever going to be any hope of creating a healthier and more active society, then this is an outlook that desperately needs to be changed on a national level.

The reality is that exercise doesn't solely revolve around lifting heavy weights or running endless miles and it's definitely not all exhausting, repetitive and boring. You really need to reassess your views and understanding of what options are available and realise there's a range of possibilities to get involved in that suit all ages, abilities and fitness levels. From yoga to swimming, sports like golf or tennis, jogging, climbing or simply going for walks on a regular basis, the key to it all is finding an activity you enjoy and that you feel you can stick to it. You can even choose the environment and circumstances you feel comfortable in, from working out on your own, participating in group classes, getting involved in outdoor activities or programmes you can do at home.

I know how difficult it is to start trying to incorporate exercise into your lifestyle when mentally you have the mindset that you can't do it. Growing up I was always terrible at sports and this deterred me further from ever trying anything else, as I always believed I wouldn't be good at any form of physical activity and automatically assumed I wouldn't find it fun either. That right there is a fundamental flaw in itself, as the belief that you have to be amazing just to give it a go is simply far too much pressure. When instead the onus should be placed on doing it because it's fun, enjoyable and good for your health, not to show off or prove something. This mindset and belief isn't just holding people back in regards to exercise either. It's a limitation people are placing on themselves for a whole array of areas and activities throughout life, preventing them from trying new things or pushing their comfort zones.

The honest truth is the first few times entering a gym I felt massively out of place and embarrassed, feeling like everyone was judging me due to how clueless and out of shape I was. In fact, I even had a few occasions where I went in and left due to it being too busy, telling myself I'll go back later when there are less people around so that I could do my workout properly. But the truth is no one actually cares. Everyone is there for the same reason and everyone knows we all had to start somewhere. Obviously you may still get the occasional person who judges others due to their own insecurities, but they are few and far between and those negative emotions you feel are simply based on your mindset of self-doubt, which is natural when you question whether or not you are capable of doing something. Believe it or not, I have actually found that the fitness community is extremely friendly, helpful and supportive of new people trying to embark on a journey to a healthier, more active lifestyle, which is the complete opposite to my original perception. I have found its actually common practice for people to go out of their way to help those who ask for assistance. But just like with everything else in this book, it is all about making up your mind that this is what you want, and being determined that you will do it, as once you take the first steps, everyday will become easier.

"Physical fitness is not only one of the most important keys to a healthy body, it is the basis of dynamic and creative intellectual activity."
- John F. Kennedy

Ways to become more active

As with all parts of this programme, the first steps to incorporating change are the hardest, and doing too much too soon can deter you further. Instead the aim should be to start small so you can build up your confidence, as you will no doubt find that you are far more capable than you give yourself credit for. Many people worry they don't know what to do, how long to do it for, or fear they will get injured and often use these reasons to justify to themselves as to why they shouldn't even bother trying. But while these are all legitimate concerns, they are also merely excuses. There are so many resources for support out there that no matter your level or understanding, you can find ways to ease into adding exercise to your lifestyle. Even if you are injured or have a disability, there are ways you can work around it, it may just require some planning or thought to determine the best route to take.

To help put your mind at rest, I thought I would go through a few activities you could engage in, along with situations you may find yourself in and how you can resolve the barriers you may face. I have tried to divide the insights up between various different options, but due to the sheer amount of potential activities, this is very much a generalised overview. Because of that, you will find that these ideas definitely overlap, and the strategies covered will in one way or another be applicable to a variety of other activities you may decide to try. Again this has been done to get you thinking, and it will be up to you to take the ideas discussed and apply them directly to whatever it is you decide to do.

Joining a gym

If joining a gym for the first time is the route you decide to go, then I highly advise you ask for help on form (the way to safely perform an exercise with correct posture and movement) and technique, rather than simply guessing. Every gym floor is scattered with personal trainers and members of staff whose job is to help and advise on how to use everything from weights to machines or exercise programming. Most gyms will give you a free session to talk and guide you through it all when you initially sign up, which is definitely worth attending.

There seems to be a huge misperception that personal trainers are unapproachable, scary beings you can't talk to, or whom you need to pay for simple advice such as how to use a piece of equipment, whereas the opposite is actually true. The majority of trainers got into the industry with the aim of helping people and that's exactly why they are there. I have found from my own experience working as a personal trainer that many of them are actually just as scared or nervous to approach you and offer support as you are to approach them. Believe it or not, it can actually be quite daunting standing around all day trying to build up the confidence to go and talk to people, which is why you need to get over the mindset that it's embarrassing to ask for help, or to not know what you are doing. You need to remember that the temporary moment of swallowing your pride will, in the long run, be hugely beneficial to your health and lifestyle. This is especially true when first embarking on trying to become more active, regardless of the activity chosen. The last thing you want to do is hurt or injure yourself, as this would likely just put you off and reaffirm your initial misconceptions and hesitations. It may even stop you from trying again.

Nonetheless, even when you feel more comfortable with your programme, it helps to regularly assess what you are doing, as there will always be ways to improve. YouTube is an excellent resource I often use for guides and tutorials on how to do certain exercises that take some getting used to. It's also definitely worth getting someone to film you doing the movements, as that way you can watch them back and evaluate areas you need to work on.

Walking or running

At the opposite side of the spectrum, if the direction you choose to take for increasing your physical activity is walking or running, then plan a route you know you can get through. This removes the fear of landing up stuck somewhere if you over-estimated how far you can go, then in time, you can build up to longer distances. Even if you plan a course that just goes around the block several times, if you feel up to it, you can keep going while remaining in an environment you feel safe and comfortable until you feel confident in pushing yourself further. You will find that once you have done the course a few times any negative perceptions you may have had towards the activity will disappear. Your mind will be at ease and you will be able to embrace enjoying it far more, without being anxious or overwhelmed. These feelings are common place when initially stepping outside of your comfort zone, along with potentially feeling embarrassed or uncomfortable. We all go through it and facing those challenges head on will directly help you grow as a person. What's important though is aiming to continually progress. This can be done by increasing the intensity or distance as you become more comfortable with the activity. Push for that extra lap, run that extra mile, jog instead of walk. The feeling afterwards is one of the most rewarding experiences you can have, and pushing yourself in this manner will be essential for your continued progress. Just don't try and do it all at once. Take a couple of weeks initially to get used to the activity, evaluate how you have done and then see how you can make it more of a challenge. Initially the main focus is all about developing a habit upon which you can build, so always remember, something is far better than nothing and at the start it's simply all about getting yourself into the routine of going through with it.

Yoga and classes

Yoga is another great activity that burns a surprising amount of calories. Not only that, but it's also great for your mental and physical health. There's a range of types to suit all interests and abilities, from fast to slow moving, to hot yoga, strength based training, or even classes that combine yoga elements with other meditative movements and breathing patterns such as Tai Chi. In fact, many fitness group classes which incorporate yoga and Tai Chi elements include a five-minute meditation at the end of the class, precisely to help with clearing your mind. Focusing on your breathing helps you unwind, improves your sleep and helps you be more mindful of your own body. This in itself links directly to improving your overall mindset, and if this is an area you are struggling with then engaging in this practice may be exactly what you need to relax, manage stress, and temporarily distances yourself from the challenges you faced throughout the day.

There are tonnes of classes around for all levels and interests, but if you are still uncertain, contact the instructor beforehand and let them know that while you want to try their class, you are apprehensive. They will be able to advise you on whether their class is suitable for you, as well as talk you through exactly what's involved and, if necessary, make suggestions on alternatives. This applies for any class activity, from spinning to circuits or Zumba, not just yoga. I highly advise having a look at what's on in your local area, as there will be a variety of offerings available at different gyms, leisure clubs, schools, or even village halls. But if you don't feel ready to go to a class or are short on time, you can always follow along to tutorials at home.

Yoga is something I have become really keen on over the past few years, as it's great for both injury prevention and rehabilitation. Be that as it may, I'll be the first to put my hand up and admit I initially had the misperception that it was mostly for hippies or women, but I'm willing to admit when I'm wrong. By forcing myself to push my comfort zones and enter a new environment in which I initially found myself to be massively uncomfortable in, I was able to find an activity that I actually really enjoy. As someone coming from a largely sedentary background and having developed poor posture over the years from sitting at a desk or slouching on the couch, it's great for helping my injured lower back and is also really relaxing.

Classes also have the added benefit of teaching you basic form for a variety of movements while under supervision, and without having to pay for one-to-one coaching from a personal trainer. If you are new to exercise then this could be a great way to get experience with what you are doing and improve your confidence, all while being in a fun and supportive environment.

Swimming

For those of you reading this who have health issues such as arthritis, or are trying to recover from an injury, it may be best to consider a low impact sport such as swimming. Not only is swimming great for your cardiovascular health, but it can also help ease the pain in sore joints and help extend your range of motion. I found this to be particularly true when I was trying to ease myself into exercise while rehabbing a lower back and knee injury. This was at a time when I struggled placing any pressure on my legs and because of that, was unable to partake in any form of running, cycling or weight lifting. This is the perfect example of finding an activity that's best suited to your ability, interests and health.

Taking up a sport

If you are looking for something a bit more competitive and interactive, you could always take up a sport. With just a few of the options available ranging from tennis to squash, badminton, football, volleyball or even martial arts. Playing sports is great for the simple reason that often you will land up pushing yourself far harder than normal, without even realising it and you will expose yourself to new situations and experiences, helping you meet and interact with new people, thereby pushing your comfort zones in other aspects of your life. If you are trying to find ways to manage your stress levels then these activities could aid in helping you relax, unwind, or get your mind off of life's other pressures, as walking round a golf course may be exactly what you need after a long week at work. So give it some thought, as you can either engage in these with family or friends, or you could look at what local teams and clubs are located near you.

Resistance training

While I do believe the focus should be on basing your chosen activity around practices you enjoy, there is one exception, and that is resistance training, which is also commonly referred to as strength training. There are various different activities that fall into this category, including weight lifting, using machines, or even just movements using your body weight. Although resistance training is often perceived in a negative light due to the way the industry is portrayed, it's one aspect of exercise that everyone, young or old, should be incorporating in some form into their lives. Don't misinterpret that to mean I'm saying you should be spending every day in the gym, grunting in the corner and obsessing over the size of your biceps, as that couldn't be farther from truth or what it actually entails.

There's a reason why I believe resistance training is so important, because as you get older you start to lose muscle mass and bone density, which leads to a range of issues from insulin sensitivity problems to weak bones and joints. Physically inactive people can lose as much as three to five percent muscle mass every decade after the age of 30, making them more susceptible to falls, trips and injuries, along with various age-related issues such as osteoporosis. Older people are also at an increased risk for diabetes, hypertension and other chronic diseases. By engaging in resistance training you are able to build and preserve muscle, improve balance, stamina, posture and coordination. Other health benefits include better sleep, decreased cortisol levels, higher self-confidence and an improved sense of wellbeing. It's because of this that you should be looking to both build and preserve as much muscle mass as you can, which is something that can be done at any age. Albeit, it's obviously easier when you are younger, but don't let that deter you, as it's always better to start late rather than never.

If you don't have access to a gym or if the weight section scares, intimidates or simply doesn't appeal to you, don't feel like it's an activity you are excluded from or can't partake in. This type of exercise can easily be done at home with the use of some cheap dumbbells, or even body weight training (which is basically doing exercises like squats or push-ups with just your body and no equipment).

One misperception I need to put to rest is the fact that if you are female and follow a weightlifting routine that it will cause you to look 'bulky', as this couldn't be farther from the truth. When you look at the biology behind it all, women have far less testosterone than men do in their bodies, and because of that, it takes them far longer to build muscle. Not only that, but even when they do it doesn't make them look like a bodybuilder, as increased muscle mass often goes hand in hand with reduced body fat percent, thereby creating the more 'toned' look that so many people desire. The women you see who fit the misperceived image have either spent years rigorously training, or have achieved this look through the use of performance enhancing drugs. So don't worry, lifting up a dumbbell is not going to drastically change the way you look overnight, and you have nothing to fear by adding resistance training into your lifestyle.

The 'Become a Better You' workouts

To make adding this activity into your life easier I have put together a couple of workouts you can complete at home, either using body weight training or dumbbells. If this way of exercising is new to you, then I advise starting with the body weight routine for a few weeks and then progressing onto the dumbbell routine when you feel more comfortable. Don't worry if many if not all of these movements are something that are new to you, as a few years ago I would have felt just as confused. That's why I have recorded several tutorials on how to safely and effectively perform these movements, and you can access them at:

www.tailoredlifestyles.co.uk/workouts.

Body weight training

Circuit one:
Squats
Push-ups (on knees if needed)
Plank (hold for 30 seconds or however long possible)
Step ups/high knees/running on the spot

Circuit two:
Lunges
Dips (using a bed or table)
Crunches
Mountain climbers (both legs count as one rep, so 24 total)

Dumbbell training

Circuit one:

Dumbbell goblet squats

Push-ups (on knees if needed)

Plank (hold for 30 seconds or however long possible)

Step ups/high knees/running on the spot

Circuit two:

Dumbbell lunges

Overhead triceps push

Bent over row or renegade row

Crunches

Circuit three:

Dumbbell goblet squats

Dumbbell shoulder press

Alternating bicep curl

Mountain climbers (both legs count as one rep, so 24 total)

These are great introductory plans that can be done anywhere from your home, to a gym or hotel room. Best of all, they can be completed at your own pace. If doing the dumbbell plan make sure you choose a weight that you feel comfortable with, while still being challenging and not too heavy.

How to do them

To perform these circuits, you have a few options depending on your fitness level or preference. Initially I'd advise starting with option one, and then progressing accordingly as you become more comfortable:

Option one:

Perform 12 repetitions or the stated time of an exercise, rest for 30 seconds, then move onto the next. At the end of each circuit rest one to two minutes before starting the next circuit and repeat if possible.

Option two:

Perform 12 repetitions or the stated time of each exercise in circuit one, one after the other with as little rest in between as possible, rest for one to two minutes and then move onto the next circuit. Repeat if possible.

Option three:

Set a timer for seven minutes and run through circuit one, doing 12 repetitions or the stated time before moving onto the next exercise. Complete as many rounds as possible within the time frame, rest two minutes then do the same with the next circuit.

Regardless of your preferences, ability or goals, you can easily find a way to incorporate resistance training into your lifestyle and see substantial benefit from doing so. Alternative you could look at some types of yoga with postures that incorporate aspects of resistance training, as they are a great way to build a solid foundation and preserve muscle.

When and how often should you do it?

Because these are full body workouts you need to ensure you take a day off in between doing them to allow your body to properly rest and recover. The reason why this is so essential is because during these 'rest days' your body is able to repair itself and build new muscle. To see the most benefit from these activities you ideally want to be completing them three times a week, aiming for a minimum of two. None of the above plans will take more than 20 to 30 minutes, and you can do them whenever you can fit them in. Whether that's in the morning, after work, or even at lunch time, is completely up to you. With that being said though, it's best to try and develop some form of routine, where you aim to complete them at regular and consistent times, in order to develop the habit.

Resistance training and weight goals

Resistance training is hugely beneficial for both weight loss and maintenance, due to the influence it has on increasing your muscle mass. Since muscle requires more energy, your metabolism increases because your body burns more calories on a daily basis, even at rest. On top of that, you respond better to insulin, keeping your levels more stable and avoiding metabolic syndrome, which is the name given to a group of risk factors associated with developing cardiovascular disease, type 2 diabetes, or strokes.

Conclusion

This is very much a limited list of potential activities and you can no doubt think of others. But hopefully it has at least got you to think about some of the avenues you can pursue, along with ways in which to get yourself to push your comfort zones and overcome any potential obstacles that may prevent you from getting started.

"The greater the obstacle, the more glory in overcoming it."
- Molière

Overcoming barriers

Now that you know why exercising is so important, have a better idea about how to choose an activity to engage in and how to get started, it's time to shift the focus to other issues that may be standing in your way. When it comes to change, we all have barriers stopping us from pursuing certain aspects within our lives, whether that's becoming more active, eating healthier, pushing ourselves in social situations, or even attempting to take the next step in our career. Regardless of who you are there will always be elements of self-doubt, confidence and anxiety. But again, breaking through them is all about pushing your comfort zones and finding ways around parts of your life that are holding you back. The easiest way to overcome them is to determining exactly what they are, as this is the first step in actively making progress. By recognising what barriers you face, you can work out a plan or strategy in which to deal with them. Thereby not only making the entire process easier, but also making it far more likely you will be able to overcome them, as you will be better prepared as and when they arise.

For now, we will be focusing on barriers related to exercise, along with strategies you can use to overcome then. You will however find that many of the issues discussed can and do apply to other issues as well, and we will be returning to this topic later, looking at strategies related to overcoming barriers in regards to eating healthier.

Time

When conducting research for this book I spoke to people from a wide variety of backgrounds, from nurses to business professionals and stay at home parents, with the aim of uncovering the biggest barriers they faced in regards to improving their wellbeing. The issue of "time" topped the list as the most frequently mentioned factor, stopping them from not only becoming more active, but also paying attention to other aspects of their health. The honest truth is there will never be a right time to focus on your wellbeing, which is why there's no way around it, if you truly want to get healthier then you need to find a way to shift priorities or change your routine to fit it in. Whether that means freeing up time in the evening, working out at lunch time, or getting up slightly earlier in the morning, the small inconvenience can help avoid a whole host of pain and suffering in the long run. At first it may feel like a sacrifice, or something you really don't want to do, which is why so many people use this excuse to convince themselves that they are simply too busy to find the time. Yet the Nelson Report released statistics saying the average American watches more than 34 hours of TV a week! That is around five hours per day, and these viewing averages remain at high levels for countries throughout the Western World. For many, the 'I don't have time' excuse is actually a 'I'm more comfortable in front of the TV and don't want to move' excuse.

I have lost count of how many people I have worked with who have inevitably admitted that they could find time for focusing on their health if they really wanted to. It's just not on their list of priorities and the first challenge they face is overcoming this mindset. If that sounds like you then the good news is with a little thought and preparation, this can be done in a way that fits into your lifestyle and routine, without having to make endless sacrifices or completely change who you are. Whether you are trying to become more active, improve your diet, or any other aspect of your life, when time is a barrier, planning is key. You plan most other things in your life and your health needs to initially be treated in exactly the same way. Like many changes in this book, to start with it's all about making the healthy option the easy option, creating cues and pushing yourself to go through with it. Luckily though there are strategies you can use to do exactly that.

Strategies for getting round the barrier of time

Planning

Depending on how far ahead your schedule is mapped out, I suggest having a look at your calendar and finding areas in which you either have, or can free up some time. And if you don't have a calendar, now is the time to make one! Highlight the time slot(s) where you can become more active and schedule it in as a part of your day. That way you are far less likely to cancel on yourself. Also knowing what times you can be free will help you decide whether you will be attending a class, going to the gym, or simply working out at home.

Use proper time management

If you have an extremely hectic schedule and can't free up an hour to exercise, then break it down into 30 or even 15 minute slots. Those short bursts quickly add up and this may be a good strategy if exercise is new to you, or if it's something you perceive as an action you won't enjoy. That's because it's far easier to convince yourself to face it for 15 minutes, rather than an hour.

Pack your bag the night before

That way you can go straight from work, as by the time you have gone home, changed and left to go to the gym or your class, you could probably already have been done with your workout.

Exercise at home

Exercising at home is great, as you can cut out any time spent commuting and you could do anything from yoga to circuits or weights. Just try and do it as soon as you get through the door, as all the good intentions in the world can quickly be lost as soon as you enter a comfortable environment and get tempted to just relax.

Find ways to walk more on a daily basis

As already mentioned, people often overlook the idea of walking more and if you work extremely long hours then taking breaks to go for works may be the perfect option if you have no other alternative. If you could do this on a daily basis you will quickly see the benefits of your actions and you can then focus on incorporating other activities on your off days.

Have a proper plan

If you have a proper fitness regime you can save time by training 'smarter' and ensuring you get the most value out of the time you do put to use. Ultimately 30 minutes of a properly structured workout is far more effective than an hour aimlessly bouncing around from one machine to another in a gym. However, it's best to avoid one size fits all programmes you find online as much as possible. This is because everyone responds differently, and chances are the way in which they are designed will in all likelihood not be the optimal approach for reaching your goals. Especially when you are under the added pressure of trying to make the best use of your time as possible. Having said that, if resistance training is new to you then you will see great results from starting with the plan included in this book, and then you can look to move onto a more personalised routine as you progress in the future.

Incorporate exercise into family activities

Turn those family days out into an activity that gets everyone moving, such as going for a swim, a bike ride, or even a walk. There is something for every family out there, and exercise won't feel like a chore if you are having fun and spending time with the most important people in your life.

Do as much as you can

Regardless of how committed you are, there will always be times when life gets in the way. So when this happens just try and do as much as you can, without adding further pressure on yourself to be perfect. Just remember - something is always better than nothing and over time all those positive actions will add up.

Motivation

The next most common barrier to come up during my research was a lack of motivation. Like with most new ventures, your habits have a huge influence on your motivation, which is why you need to break away from what you are comfortable with. As hard as it is at first, it may be a case of forcing yourself to find the motivation, or changing and cutting back on what you previously viewed as important to free up some time, such as the amount of TV shows you watch per week. It may not seem like it now, but if given the chance, exercise will in time become part of your routine and hopefully a part of your life that you not only enjoy, but also look forward to. This is key, as it has been proven that any activity or factor that's pleasurably sustainable will in turn decrease stress hormones and vastly improve your health, mindset and overall happiness. These benefits will inevitably make it far easier to stick to it, which is why you need to choose an activity you can see yourself enjoying. It's just like dieting, no matter how good your intentions are, if you hate doing it or view it as a form of punishment, it will never be more than a short term measure at best. That's why it's essential you properly think about and plan what you are going to do, as it's vital you are able to get over the mindset of resenting having to do it. A quote often used by successful people and originally said by Benjamin Franklin says "Fail to plan, you plan to fail", which is extremely accurate when it comes to exercise. That's because failing to plan is a recipe for disaster, as before long your motivation will quickly run dry. If however you can find an activity you at least see yourself enjoying, then there are ways to get yourself to act upon it in the initial stages before it becomes a habit.

Strategies for overcoming barriers of motivation

Accountability

I have found the easiest way to motivate and get someone to stick to something is to set up a system of accountability that holds them to the desired action. This will play a substantial role in the overall plan in the final section, but for now, here are some examples of ways install accountability:

-   Get a family member or friend to join you. Having a partner makes it harder to cancel and they can push you to exercise even at times when you are not in the mood. It can also make the experience less daunting and more fun.

-   Alternatively, if you struggle exercising alone, is there a class you could join? Regularly booking in for a class makes it far more likely you will attend, due to the inner feeling of guilt attached to cancelling that you may not experience from simply not going out for a run or to the gym on your own.

-   By using the system and measures discussed in the final section of this book.

Not knowing what you want to do

You might be thinking that no form of exercise really appeals to you and this can tie in directly with struggling to find motivation to try adding exercise to your routine. In this case, it's best to start with what you think you will most likely be able to do and stick to, or even push yourself out of your comfort zone and try a range of different activities. You may be shocked to find what you actually enjoy once you break through your negative preconception of what it actually involves. As I said before, that happened to me with yoga. Although I don't overly like classes or the slow meditation variants, I found a more cardio-based version that I can do at home.

Focus on changing your mindset

Getting into the mindset of continuously reinforcing the reasons and benefits of what you are doing can help in forming new habits. This mindset may keep you motivated or give you a push to keep going during parts of activities you don't overly enjoy, or when you feel like giving up. For example, I enjoy lifting weights and going to the gym, but like a lot of people, I find cardio beyond boring. Yet I'm able to do it due to the mindset I have that includes understanding how good it is for my health. I remind myself how good I feel afterwards, and that it's only 30 minutes of my day a couple of times a week. With this approach it really doesn't feel that bad, and I always walk away feeling glad I did it. In most cases I personally couldn't think of anything worse than going to a gym and walking on a treadmill, which is why instead I choose to plan walks around where I live. You may however be the opposite and find joining a gym with TVs or monitors on where you can still enjoy your favourite shows may be the happy medium of getting you to compromise, as you can engage in an action that's good for your health, all while still doing something you enjoy. This same goes for getting a treadmill, bike or cross trainer for your house, meaning you can use them at your own convenience or whenever works for you.

Combine exercise with other tasks or activities

You could be productive during certain activities by engaging in other tasks at the same time. For instance, you could listen to audiobooks or podcasts to help further develop your knowledge or understanding on a topic that's relevant to your life or interests. In turn, this can help counter any feelings of boredom, thereby keeping you motivated. It may also be a way around a barrier such as lack of time when it comes to progressing your career or understanding of a particular subject. For instance, I tend to listen to podcasts on everything from health, to business, discussions of world events or simply comedy. I have found this helps with conducting research, gets my mind off the activity at hand, and expands my understanding on various topics I would have had to look into at a later date. Therefore, saving me from having to find time elsewhere. Listening to them also helps the time pass quicker, as I'm not thinking 'one song finished, only nine more to go', a train of thought I often fall into when just listening to music, inevitably causing time to drag.

Final thoughts

Hopefully the strategies mentioned above will give you some ideas as to what you could try and incorporate, and you will no doubt be able to think of others that are specific to you, your lifestyle, routine and chosen activity. Some of them may seem like common sense or too simple, but trust me, they can and will make a huge difference and may be the deciding factor when you are on the fence as to whether or not to go through with the activity.

Even when your chosen activities are part of your routine, there will always be days when you are tired or feel less motivated than others. But one thing you will find is that no matter how much you have to force yourself to go through with it, you will never regret having done so. What I have found especially true is on days when you feel tired and fatigued, pushing yourself to exercise invigorates you. There have been many mornings where I have walked into a gym, not in the mood and debating whether or not I should have stayed in bed, only to feel revitalised a few minutes later with a sudden burst of energy. Those times often turn into the best work out of the week and give me a feeling of positivity that directly transitions into all other tasks throughout the rest of the day. On those days, you walk away with a feeling of accomplishment and are proud of yourself that you pushed through, especially when it would have been far easier to just go back to sleep or retreat straight to the sofa.

"Exercise is King, nutrition is Queen, put them together and you have got a kingdom."

- Jack LaLanne

Pre and Post work out nutrition

One thing you need to consider when exercising is what to consume before and after your workout to ensure you fuel your body with the nutrients it requires to perform and recover. This increases in importance depending on the duration, intensity and type of activity you do. For example, pre and post work out nutrition plays a vital role in resistance training, long distance running or other high intensity sports, whereas it's not really an aspect you need to worry about when engaging in lower impact activities such as walking, yoga or moderate swimming, as they don't place anywhere near as much strain on your body.

Pre-workout nutrition

When considering pre-workout nutrition, it's easy to make the mistake of not realising that it can take your body several hours to metabolise the nutrients you consume. Therefore, depending on the size of the meal, if you don't give it adequate time to digest, you may not actually see any benefit from what you eat beforehand.

It's important to remember that eating too much can lead to feeling bloated or sick, whereas failing to eat can lead to reduced energy and low blood sugar levels, which can cause light-headedness or fatigue. I say 'can', as everyone responds differently and as with most things in health and fitness, there is no one-size-fits-all correct answer. Because of that, what you eat will largely be dependent on a combination of personal preference, what foods you enjoy, outside circumstances and how your body reacts to the food. It may very well come down to a trial and error process to determine what is best for you.

But before we get into that, for a brief moment let's get a little 'sciencey'.

If you have heard anyone talk about 'fuelling their body', then you may have heard the terms glucose and glycogen thrown around. To simplify it as much as possible, glucose is basically what provides you with energy throughout the day and is obtained when the carbohydrates you consume are broken down into sugars within your body. When the body senses you have excess glucose, it uses a process called glycogenesis to convert it into glycogen, which it then stores in muscle and liver tissues as a fuel reserve for later use. When you exercise, you deplete the glucose in your blood faster, causing your body to turn to your glycogen stores and convert them back into glucose through a process called glycolysis. This is why it's important to provide your body with the correct nutrients to keep your levels topped up, as well as to restore them when depleted. One of the risks of not having sufficient reserves is that exercise can lead to muscle loss, as the body is forced to resort to entering a catabolic state where it breaks down muscle for energy. However, this is primarily a concern in anaerobic exercise (activities that are high intensity or revolve around short, intense bursts such as weightlifting), and not something you should be concerned with if you have eaten properly beforehand.

Protein

If you look into it enough, you will find people on both sides of the argument as to whether or not you need protein before exercise. They will disagree as to whether or not it leads to less muscle breakdown, or whether it furthers muscle growth. However, what is often not taken into consideration is the fact that it takes your body several hours to ingest a large meal (between two to six hours) and because of that, what it comes down to is when and what you last ate. For that reason, if you had a sizeable amount of protein within an hour or two before exercising then further amounts aren't necessary. However, if it has been several hours before your last intake or the previous amount eaten was relatively small (less than 20 grams), then consuming 20 to 40 grams would be beneficial to spike plasma amino acid levels and begin protein synthesis before training.

Carbohydrates

While the importance of protein is often disputed, the ability of carbohydrates to improve performance is undeniable. When consumed before exercise, carbohydrates provide your body with additional fuel, giving you more energy, and for most people, allowing them to push themselves harder than they would have without it. It's for this reason that you should be aiming to consume a reasonable amount before and after your training to help your body with both energy and recovery.

Let's look at what to consider depending on your time frames:

If you are eating around 30 minutes before exercise your aim should be to consume a 100 to 200 calorie snack that can be quickly absorbed by your body. Depending on the type of training (especially with resistance training), it may be beneficial to ensure this meal is a mix of both protein and carbohydrates, aiming for around 25 to 50 grams carbohydrates, and 20 to 40 grams protein.

To put that into perspective, a medium size banana is around 25 grams of carbohydrate and 20 grams of protein is around half a chicken breast, a small pot of Greek yoghurt, or one scoop of protein powder.

Some examples of what to eat 30 minutes before:
- Fruits such as bananas, pineapple, mangoes or watermelon. (Can be eaten on their own, or in the form of a smoothie)
- Whey protein shake
- Fruit and yoghurt

If you are eating an hour or two, or three to four hours before exercising, then your aim should be to eat a more nutritionally balanced meal, consisting of both protein and slow release carbohydrates, with the carbohydrates making up around 50 to 60 percent of the meal. This is done in order to keep your blood sugar levels stable, and give you energy throughout the workout. While the food sources remain similar, you should look to make the meal larger depending on how long it is before your activity.

Examples of what to eat:

- Chicken and brown rice
- A bowl of whole wheat pasta with protein
- Poached eggs on whole-wheat toast
- Whole-wheat tuna/chicken sandwich
- Oatmeal and nuts with Greek yoghurt or protein powder
- Greek yoghurt and fruit
- Baked potato with beans or chicken
- An omelette
- Peanut butter and wholemeal toast

What to avoid before working out

- Sugary foods such as chocolate and candy. These cause a sugar rush and may result in a sugar crash in the middle of the workout, leading to a drop in energy or causing you to feel light-headed.
- Fried food

Fat

You may have noticed I haven't mentioned eating fat in this section and that's because I wanted to keep it as straight forward as possible. There is a huge misperception in the fitness industry that consuming fat before your workout should be avoided. This is due to the idea that since it takes your body longer to break fats down, it would also slow how quickly the carbohydrates you ingest can be put to use, which would affect whether or not they could be utilised for performance.

While in theory this makes sense, more recent studies have

proven otherwise, stating consuming fat doesn't impact nutrient utilisation and thereby concluding it's not an issue you need to be overly concerned with. While fats may not hinder performance, there are no proven benefits attributed to their use either, so whether or not you choose to include fat in your pre-workout meal is entirely up to you. Nevertheless, it's worth considering that fat can potentially lead to stomach discomfort issues. However, this is largely dependent on how your body responds, so it may be best to lean on the cautious side and keep intake on the lower end. Like I said though, don't overthink it, as some great high protein pre-workout foods such as eggs or peanut butter actually have high amounts of healthy fat in them.

Personally, if I'm going to eat one or two hours before working out, then my pre-workout meal usually consists of a bowl of oats with a banana, Greek yoghurt and a scoop of protein powder. If it's half an hour before, I usually half the amount of oats and drop the Greek yoghurt, opting for just the protein powder instead, as it's absorbed and broken down faster.

The reason why I tend to turn to these meals is simply because I mostly train in the morning, making quick breakfast foods the most convenient options.

Post workout

Along with restoring glycogen stores, the aim of post-workout nutrition is to stimulate protein synthesis so the body can properly recover and grow. This is because when you exercise, your body starts a process called proteolysis, where muscle proteins are broken down and rebuilt. While that sounds like a potentially detrimental process, it's actually important, as it relates to the body's ability to synthesise and create protein molecules. When it synthesises more than is lost, new muscle is built and vice versa.

The anabolic window

It has long been believed that after exercise there exists something called an 'anabolic window', which is a period of time when your body can best absorb and make use of nutrients you consume. Failing to do so can hinder muscle growth and recovery, which is why if you enter any gym you will no doubt find people rushing to down their protein shakes immediately after they are done, acting like it's the be all and end all of mission impossible, where every precious second counts in a desperate attempt to not lose out on any possible 'gains' or benefits.

But does it really matter?

In a way yes, but not within the time frame or to the extent many people have been led to believe. Research does indicate that eating after exercise aids in recovery and muscle repair and because of that it is beneficial regardless of the type of exercise you have taken part in. With that in mind, you should aim to consume a meal within two hours of completing your activity, as it's during this period when glycogen re-synthesis is at around 150 percent of its normal rate. Even this time frame is however disputed, with many experts arguing that the anabolic window stretches far beyond the two hour mark. The message to take away from this is that if you can't or don't want to eat immediately after your workout, then don't panic, as you won't be hindering your results. Instead, just look to have a sufficient meal as soon as you can.

How much do you need?

Studies have found that 20 grams of protein is a sufficient amount to stimulate protein synthesis in most people. However, as previously mentioned, everyone is different and this amount can fluctuate depending on your age, how intense your workout was, how much muscle mass you have or even how your hormones respond. Because of that, it's best to view 20 grams as the minimum amount and ideally you should be aiming to get around 20 to 40 grams. With carbohydrates, the general consensus is that you should be looking to take in around one gram for every kilo of bodyweight. But unless you are an athlete or training more than once a day, then there's no real rush to restore your glycogen levels, as the process will continue throughout the day. The point to take away from this all is that consuming protein is what's vital after your workout.

The meal ideas for after you exercise are pretty much exactly the same as the suggestions for what to eat a few hours prior to the activity. But if you are in a rush, you can easily get away with just having a protein shake, as that will keep you going until you can have a sufficient meal later on.

Final thoughts

Hopefully by now you have a better idea as to why it's so important that you find ways to become more active, even if it's still something you are intimidated by or not overly keen to do. If however you are still on the fence or not sold on the concept and thinking you can get away with just improving your diet, remember that no matter how healthy you eat, diet can't be used as a substitute for the health benefits gained through regular exercise. However, I've said it before and I'll say it again, on the other side of this you simply can't exercise your way out of a bad diet, no matter how hard you try. For too long, exercise has been perceived as the main contributor towards weight loss and instead it needs to be viewed as simply another tool in the process.

"It is exercise alone that supports the spirits, and keeps the mind in vigor."

- Cicero

Activity 4

Becoming more active

Earlier I listed a few ideas and examples of activities you could try, along with some ways to help you figure out how to get started. Obviously I couldn't list all available options, as the possibilities are nearly endless. Before moving on I want you to spend some time thinking about what physical activities you would most likely enjoy, along with the environment you want to do it in, and then push yourself into giving something a try.

This may entail looking online at what classes are going on around you, finding a nearby gym, looking for routines to do at home, doing the resistance training routine, or checking a local map to plan a route to go for walks or runs. The entire purpose of this relates back to the previous chapter of setting a goal, as creating a plan is a huge aspect in involved in the process. The aim is to move yourself from thinking about or wanting to do something, into the stage of actually planning it. Writing it down and committing to it will help in the first steps of going through with it.

The entire purpose of this task is to force yourself to push your comfort zones, as that will be the only way you will start becoming the best version of yourself. At this stage it's all about starting to developing healthier habits, so ideally you want to be finding ways to become more active at least three times a week. Whether that's going for a 30-minute walk three evenings a week, doing yoga at home after work or attending a gym, it all comes down to what you decide to do. You can even mix it up by engaging in a few different activities just to keep things interesting.

Pillar Three
Sleep, rest and recovery

"A man too busy to take care of his health is like a mechanic too busy to take care of his tools."
- Spanish proverb

As life becomes increasingly busier, people are continuously borrowing energy from tomorrow just to try and get through today. From longer workdays, to endless hours on social media, staying up late binge watching the latest shows, or playing video games. In the moment there always seems to be something that feels more important than prioritising time to rest and recover, making it no wonder as to why so many of us are always feeling burnt out or exhausted. The problem is we are always on the go, constantly burning the candle at both ends, barely stopping to think, let alone rest. High quality sleep seems to have become a thing of the past, and it's now often seen as a long forgotten luxury, as we are continually pushing our bodies to the limit.

The problem is a lack of sleep has been found to raise the risk of everything from obesity to depression, diabetes, hypertension, cancer, reduced quality of life, lower productivity and increased rates of mortality. You will often read stories of people falling asleep behind the wheel or at work, causing everything from medical and occupational errors, to car crashes or industrial accidents. Without proper rest everything from your mindset to your concentration and immune system suffer, which is why it's absolutely essential you learn to listen when your body tells you what it needs, as the signs of when to slow down become abundantly clear. Part of the problem is it's too easy to turn to anything that offers a glimpse of hope of getting through the day. From coffee to energy drinks, pills or sugar-filled snacks and these billion dollar industries are forever finding new ways to supply products to a market begging for a solution to their lack of energy, completely unaware of the long-term damage they are causing to their health. Not only from the strain caused by a lack of recovery, but also from the high sugar, processed and chemical filled substances found within these products.

The introduction discussed how all the aspects contributing to your wellbeing are interrelated, from your mindset to nutrition and activity levels, along with how neglecting one area can impact performance in everything else. Well getting sufficient rest and recovery is the glue that holds it all together, as it influences everything from your mood, to your energy levels, recovery from exercise, athletic performance, food choices, concentration and ability to function properly on a day-to-day basis. Not only that, but your memory gets worse, you have more difficulty absorbing and learning new things, become worse at problem solving, and suffer from increased inflammation. Meaning that ignoring the warning signs of sleep deprivation and exhaustion has a huge impact on your overall wellbeing and your capability to cope with your job.

Several studies on large populations of adults have found that getting seven hours of sleep a night can be just as important for health as nutrition, exercise and management of stress, yet it's often the area that garners the least focus or attention in the health and fitness industry. Maybe it's down to being viewed as less exciting or glamorous, as 'get a good night's sleep' is hardly a marketable concept and it's far easier to sell someone on some 'revolutionary' new diet or training plan, than to simply say they need to take a step back, find some time to relax or go to bed earlier. We are all guilty of sacrificing sleep over something that seems more important and while from time to time you may be able to get away with it, in the grand scheme of things the only way you will be able to make any progress with your new, healthier habits, is by finding ways to implement proper balance. The development of my dad's cancer is a prime example of failure to achieve this balance, as he was working 14-hour days, stressed beyond belief, ignoring his diet and taking little to no time to rest or recover, and regularly getting less than five to six hours sleep a night. I know you are probably thinking that this won't happen to you. But just remember that neither you nor I is invincible.

"Sleep is that golden chain that ties health and our bodies together."
- Thomas Dekker

Sleep

You will often hear that adults should be aiming to get eight hours of sleep a night and while this is a good general guideline, recommendations by the National Sleep Foundation suggest that this is more of a generalisation, and just like anything else, the exact amount needed can vary from person to person. Their conclusion is that the ideal amount to avoid sleep deprivation can vary from anywhere between seven to nine hours a night and although it has been found that some people are able to function on less, it isn't recommended that you go below a minimum of six hours per night. Yet that's an amount that people from around the world are regularly failing to reach and there have been a wide range of studies on sleep habits in America, with statistics showing as much as 70 percent of the population don't get enough rest. More than 40 percent of people are getting less than six hours a night and this is a huge increase from the 1940s, where it was only 11 percent of the population.

What's more worrying still is that statistics have shown that around 40 million Americans suffer from a sleep disorder, with a further 20 million experiencing occasional issues, so it's no surprise to find that a lack of sleep is a huge contributing factor to increasing levels of obesity and chronic diseases. It has even been found that adults with poor sleep habits are 55 percent more likely to be obese, whereas children are 89 percent! Shift workers such as fire-fighters or nurses seem to be even worse off, as they have been shown to be at an even higher risk, as their irregular sleep patterns increase the chances of developing heart disease, diabetes and cancer.

When you sleep your body conducts a range of processes, from producing hormones to repairing tissue and aiding with recovery. During this time the brain produces enzymes to detoxify poisons and chemicals that have built up throughout the day, from air pollution and inhaled fumes, to pesticides found on food. When you rest you give your body the opportunity to not only repair damage, but also begin the next day with fresh DNA, antioxidants, mitochondria and detoxification pathways. For people who are physically active, partaking in regular exercise or work in manual labour, sleep is an essential part of recovery, as it's during this time that the body both repairs and develops new muscle, together with aiding in healing injuries and damage caused. It's because of this that failure to have ample rest can often lead to reduced performance, as by neglecting recovery you are reducing your body's ability to optimally perform its functions, and in turn this can have a massively detrimental impact in preventing you from achieving both your body and fitness goals. Just like you can't out-exercise a bad diet, you can't perform properly without sufficient recovery either.

There are however solutions and strategies you can incorporate into your daily or weekly routine in order change, reduce or even prevent these conditions, many of which we will be going into later in this section. As with most things in this book, one of the main focuses is all about learning to listen to your body and mind, seeing how it responds and then adapting accordingly. This is because everyone is different and because of that will be influenced by a variety of factors, from genes to age, lifestyle choices or even their surrounding environment. That's why for optimal health your aim should be to regularly get the right amount of rest needed specifically for you. One way to determine what the amount of rest you personally need is to go to bed without setting an alarm, an exercise appropriate to do when you have an extended period of time off, such as a holiday. This will lead to your body naturally waking up when it has had sufficient rest, and from there you can judge how much you actually need on a daily basis. However, be aware that if you have had long periods of insufficient rest, the first couple of days may result in you sleeping for longer in order to catch up, so you can expect fluctuations from one end of the week to the other. You may find that as your body is used to being in a routine, that you wake up at your usual time, so it may take a few days for it to settle. I know this activity is not always possible, especially when you are highly stressed or simply unable to take time off, but it is an example of a way in which you can learn to listen to your body.

Earlier you read about how stress leads to increased levels of cortisol and epinephrine and how failure to get the levels under control can have a huge influence on your health. Out of all the strategies used to lower these levels, getting proper sleep is by far the most effective, as it aids in digesting stress hormones by placing the body in the prime state to metabolise them. On the flip side of this, a loss of sleep can elevate stress levels further, due to the negative impact feelings of exhaustion place on your mindset, and research has even shown that sleep deprivation can lead to an increase in cortisol levels the following evening. This is an issue because our bodies use a clever system to regulate cortisol levels throughout the day, and as the day progresses cortisol levels generally tend to be lowered in a constant and regular manner, often knows as 'diurnal rhythm'. Through this process our body is able to keep levels low in the evening, which in turn allows for a regular sleeping pattern. On top of affecting cortisol levels, evidence shows that a lack of sleep has a direct effect on the body's resistance and sensitivity to insulin. This is hugely problematic, as it affects the body's ability to both store and burn fat, further leading to an increase in the risk of type 2 diabetes.

It doesn't just stop there though, as sleep is massively influential on both weight loss and weight gain. This is due to the various different processes that take place when you rest and how optimally they perform is directly affected by both the quality and quantity of the rest that you get. While you are asleep your body continuously burns calories throughout the night, using energy for everything from growth to repair. Because this takes place during a period where food has not been consumed for several hours, the body turns to burning fat stores as fuel, and most of the body's growth hormones are produced during this time.

Various studies have linked lack of sleep to higher levels of body fat and in order to see the correlation between the two, researchers at the University of Chicago placed ten overweight adults on a calorie restricted diet for two weeks, divided them into two groups and assigned one group to sleep eight and a half hours a night and the other for five and a half hours. The findings showed that over the two-week period, the group that slept eight and a half hours per night lost 55 percent more fat and 60 percent less muscle than the group that only slept five and a half hours. They also found that the group who got more rest experienced less feelings of hunger throughout the day, even though they were placed in the same calorie deficit.

Furthermore, sleep deprivation changes the way we think and feel about food, with various studies linking a lack of rest to making poor food choices the following day. This is due to an increase in the production of the hunger hormone ghrelin, often causing cravings for sugar and carbohydrates when you are tired in an attempt to get more energy and making it more likely that you will give into temptation or binge. If these challenges weren't hard enough as it is in this state, you also face decreased levels of leptin, the hormone that sends signals from the stomach to the brain letting it know when you are full, which in turn can lead to over eating. These two hormones being off balance plays a huge role influencing weight loss and weight gain in regards to a lack of sleep, with insufficient rest directly influencing not only the quantity, but the quality of what we choose to consume. In fact, in 2012 a study by the Mayo Clinic found that people who got 80 minutes less sleep than usual consumed on average an extra 550 calories on the following day!

With sleep deprivation causing so many issues to both our bodies and our minds, it is vital we take the time to recharge our batteries in order to keep up with our full on, faced paced lives. This part of your wellbeing isn't just about sleep though, as its essential you find ways to relax and blow off some steam. Doing so is a vital part of recovery and hugely important to clear your mind of all the pressure and negativity you face on a daily basis.

"The time to relax is when you don't have time for it."
- Sydney J. Harris

Rest and recovery

Just like with managing stress, I know you are probably thinking it's easy for me to sit here and say you need to sleep or rest more, as chances are with how hectic your life is you rarely get time to yourself, let alone have extra hours to lie around or go to bed earlier. The harsh reality is for many people it simply isn't possible to make drastic changes in overhauling their routines. After all, they work long hours, with an ever-growing list of priorities and commitments to tend to when they finish, often meaning sleep is the area that needs to be sacrificed in order to get it all done. While in a perfect world you would be able to reorganise your priorities so you can rest more, if it simply isn't possible, then for the sake of your health you need to at least find ways to relax and give your body a break, even if it means just squeezing in 10 to 15 minutes for yourself everyday, wherever you can. I know that doesn't sound like much, but again it's all about looking for ways to make small gradual changes, and you could use this time to do anything from go for a walk, fit in a short workout, mediate or even just lie down, take a break and relax.

For years I suffered from pretty severe insomnia, regularly taking an hour or two of lying in bed, restlessly tossing and turning trying to fall asleep. Even when I finally did the sleep I got was never of good quality or uninterrupted, as I'd wake up every hour or so throughout the night. Not only was it frustrating, but it was equally exhausting. I was always tired, low on energy and looking back I can clearly see how much of an impact it had on my quality of life. I would regularly go to bed exhausted, only to suddenly feel wide-awake, my mind racing with thoughts and ideas. It seemed the harder I tried to fight it and stop my mind from racing the worse it got, and my inability to manage my stress or take time to unwind was meaning I was stuck in this never ending cycle. One day I finally decided I had had enough and couldn't go on like that anymore, so I set about actively trying to find ways to change. I found several strategies that when incorporated into my daily routine worked for me in easing those problems, along with several others that have been proven to work, and will be discussed in the upcoming paragraphs.

"There is virtue in work and there is virtue in rest. Use both and overlook neither."

- Alan Cohen

Strategies for improving sleep, rest and recovery

Proper sleep hygiene and nightly rituals can have a huge impact on not only how much rest you get, but also the quality that you achieve. Once again, it's all about finding what you enjoy and works for you, so try some of these out and see how you respond, as if needed you can always adapt them accordingly.

Create a bedtime routine

Often when you lie in bed at night, your mind is still fully active thinking about the day's events and activities, along with all the stress and pressure you are currently facing. To avoid this, you need to take some time to relax and unwind, so that you can separate yourself from the thoughts relating to these circumstances. That's why it's essential you develop a ritual your body learns to associate with down time and getting ready to rest. Anything from 30 minutes to two hours before bed try to move yourself into this state of mind. Turn off all electronic devices, stop checking your email, read a book, meditate, do yoga, or any other activity you find helps you relax and prepare your body for sleep. The aim of this time should be to avoid stressful or stimulating circumstances that can lead to elevated cortisol levels, so aim to keep yourself in a calm and quiet environment, with minimal outside interference or noise.

Keep your bedroom just for sleeping

Your body builds up associations with repeated actions and habits, which is why it's vital you get into the mindset of recognising that when you are in bed, it's time to sleep. By keeping watching TV, reading or eating to a separate room or area, you can consciously tell your brain that the bedroom is for resting, and therefore you don't send mixed signals to your body. I used to make this mistake all the time, every night lying in bed watching TV, and one of the best decisions I made was to remove the TV from my bedroom. Shortly after doing so I had a far easier time falling asleep, and started sleeping for longer durations without waking up.

Have consistent times to sleep and wake up

If possible, aim to go to bed and wake up at the same time everyday. That way your body will develop an association between certain times of the day with rest and help you adapt to a routine. In order to keep your body's internal clock regulated you may need to force yourself to get up at the same time everyday (I'm sorry, but that means weekends as well). I know it's tempting to try and sleep in on nights of restless sleep, but missioning through for a few days may be the best way to get yourself adjusted to a new routine, otherwise you will simply be stuck going round in circles, as nothing ever settles down.

Change your environment to be sleep conducive

Find ways to make sure your bedroom is as dark, quiet and comfortable a temperature as possible, with being cool preferential to overly warm. Put up black out curtains, or if necessary buy an eye mask and some earplugs. Anything that helps stop you from being disturbed, or minimises distractions and interruptions.

Stop looking at screens

Using smartphones, tablets, computers and watching TV can massively influence your ability to fall asleep, as they emit a blue light that suppresses the release of the sleep-regulating hormone melatonin. That's why it's best to cut off their use at least 30 minutes before bed, as this will help stop any interference they may cause. This is probably the strategy that had the biggest impact for me, and by implementing an "electronics off" rule I was finally able to ease and relax my mind. Before it was a daily occurrence where checking emails and social media before bed would send me straight back into 'work mode', as it reawakened my mind, causing me to think about everything from what I had done that day, to my never ending to do list or tasks I needed to get done. This in turn directly contributed to causing my over active imagination at night, and why I spent hours on end tossing and turning, just trying to fall asleep. In hindsight it's such an obvious causation and necessary change, but at the time I was completely oblivious to the effect this action was truly having on my health.

Implementing this rule can reduce unnecessary distractions, and frees up time you can dedicate to other activities instead. In fact, this could be exactly the point in your day where you can make time to take 30 minutes for yourself. Initially it will take some sticking to and conscious effort to break the bad habit of always turning to your device, as in many cases it will be a gut reaction or instinct that you act upon without even thinking about it. But as with developing all new habits, with some perseverance, after a while it will just become the norm. Just remember, that email or social media status will still be there in the morning and it's not worth sacrificing those few extra hours of sleep for checking it right away.

Don't (or do?) workout late at night

Everyone is different, so this point is simply a generalisation that will depend entirely on your routine and the way in which your body responds to exercise. But for some people, working out before bed can stop them from getting proper rest, due to the elevated cortisol levels and heightened level of energy brought on by the activity. That's why ideally you want to aim to finish up at least three hours before you plan to sleep, as that way you allow these levels to stabilise and return to normal.

With that being said though, there is a chance that this will have the complete opposite effect, causing you to just want to go home and pass out, meaning it will just be a case of listening to your body and seeing how you respond.

This however only applies to intense exercise, whereas activities such as gentle yoga or light stretching can actually help you relax and unwind, making them ideal practices to incorporate into your evening routine.

Have a bath

After a long day having a hot bath may be exactly what you need to unwind. The hot water helps soothe and relax your muscles, aiding in recovery and increasing body temperature, which can prepare a tense body for falling asleep. Having a bath improves blood circulation and lowers blood pressure, therefore reducing side effects of stress, reduces headaches, moisturises your skin, helps reduce cold symptoms and brings about peace of mind. If you want to make this time even more relaxing, then look to incorporate Epsom salts. While their health benefits are debated, it's claimed they contribute to everything from relaxing the nervous system, to soothing muscle pain, healing cuts, curing skin problems, drawing toxins out the body, along with treating colds and congestion. It certainly can't hurt to try them, even if all they do is bring about a placebo effect.

Reduce caffeine intake

Everywhere you look people are relying on caffeine to help get them through the day, and while it may help for short term burst of energy, it could be having a huge influence on your ability to both fall and stay asleep. That's because caffeine is a stimulant and depending on your body's response, it can take over six hours for the effects to clear from your system. Try cutting intake off from lunch time/mid-afternoon and see if it has any positive effect.

Reduce alcohol intake

While alcohol may help you fall asleep, much like caffeine it can influence the quality of rest you get. This is due to its stimulant nature, and it can often cause you to wake up more frequently throughout the night. Reducing intake can help with getting uninterrupted sleep, and you could replace your night cap with another soothing drink instead.

Try camomile tea

Camomile tea has been used for centuries as a sleep aid, as it produces anti-anxiety effects and helps calm the nervous system. While studies have debated its direct influence on improving sleep, the simple practice of making tea, along with a soothing hot drink and its smell can clear your mind and help you unwind. Try having a cup around 30 minutes before going to bed.

Try a warm cup of milk with honey and vanilla extract

Having warm milk before bed combined with honey and vanilla extract has a range of benefits that not only help you fall asleep, but keep you asleep as well. The warm milk helps with raising your body temperature, helping you relax, while making you sleepy and calm. The honey and vanilla extract help with boosting levels of melatonin, which is what regulates the cycles in which you sleep and wake. Try having a cup of warm milk with one to two teaspoons of honey and a few drops of vanilla extract shortly before going to bed.

Ensure you are not deficient in essential nutrients

Deficiencies in certain nutrients have been proven to contribute to sleep related issues, with a lack of magnesium linked to insomnia, low levels of potassium leading to difficulties staying asleep and vitamin D causing excessive daytime sleepiness.

If necessary you can increase your intake through use of supplements, but ideally you should aim to get them through diet and a change in lifestyle choices:

Magnesium can be found in a range of leafy vegetables, nuts, seeds and legumes, and some good sources include spinach, soybeans, quinoa, sunflower seeds and almonds, along with fish such as halibut and mackerel.

Potassium rich foods include bananas, sweet potatoes, tomatoes, beets, beans, milk, fish and yoghurt.

Vitamin D is probably the nutrient people are most likely to be deficient in, especially by those who have limited access to sunshine or spend the majority of their days indoors. Your body naturally makes vitamin D when it's exposed to the sun, but you can increase your intake levels through consuming more fatty fish, egg yolks, mushrooms, cheese and other dairy products.

Meditate

Meditation is a practice used around the world to help with everything from managing stress to thinking through important decisions, regaining focus, clarity, or simply to relax. It may actually be exactly what you need in your routine after a long day, and I highly advise you give it a chance. We will be looking at a simple meditation technique you can use over the following pages.

What now?

These strategies should give you some ideas of actions you can incorporate into your daily routine and as you can see, none of them are daunting, overwhelming, inconvenient or time consuming. However, they all have the potential to have a huge influence on your ability to rest and relax. Just like a lot of the other strategies discussed throughout this book, this is very much a limited list and I'm sure you can think of other changes or actions that would directly apply to you. Finding this balance will directly spill over into improving your mindset, recovery and nutrition, which is why I highly advise you take some time to evaluate your life on the whole, so that you can determine where and how you can fit these changes in.

"It's a good idea always to do something relaxing prior to making an important decision in your life."
- Paulo Coelho

Rest and relaxation techniques

In addition to all of these strategies to improve your environment and create a relaxing bedtime routine, there are a couple of other techniques you can use to relax yourself further. These may be particularly useful to incorporate, especially during times of heightened stress, or when you are having issues with getting rest.

Breathing technique to help with falling asleep

For people who struggle falling asleep, this breathing technique can be used to help relax and lower your heart rate until you slowly drift off:

- Start by counting to four as you slowly breath in, repeating the four count as you breath out.
- Repeat this action three to four times.
- Increase to a five count, then six, then seven, repeating four times before increasing.
- As your breaths become deeper, your heart rate will continue to slow. Ensure the entire time you are trying to concentrate solely on your breathing, letting go of all other feelings and emotions filling your head, as this will bring about the soothing effect you are aiming for.

My mom actually swears by this method and she is the one who got me to start using it. As a medical professional, she regularly has long stressful days, which directly spills over into issues sleeping. That's why she now uses this method every night and so far has never made it to reaching a count of seven.

Meditation

Research has linked meditation to everything from reducing stress to handling inner distractions such as worries, cravings and desires, in addition to outer distractions such as smells, sights and sounds. It can help people clear their minds, lose weight, quit smoking, stay sober and give them strength in times they need willpower. You may have even heard tales of how people have used it to 'find themselves', or have grand epiphanies on life changing decisions that finally brings them inner peace, clarity or some other dribble about greatness. Many of the world's most successful individuals practice meditation, and it seems like everyone who is anyone has added it to their routine. Which raises the question as to whether or not it really is an effective practice, or merely just another overhyped fad.

I'll be honest, I have always been really sceptical about meditation, thinking the whole idea was pretty stupid and definitely not for me. This thinking was even reaffirmed when I got dragged along to a meditation class, as all my thoughts, prejudgments and fears came true. It was run by a weird man in a loose, flowery top and what looked like pyjama bottoms, in an attic room, with a screaming kid in the background. The entire experience was ridiculous, I hated every second and it definitely wasn't what I needed to even remotely change my mind. I remember leaving thinking how glad I was it was over and how I would never be doing that again.

But in my exhausted desire to finally get some rest, I decided I was at the point where I was willing to give anything that offered the slightest glimpse of hope a try, so I decided to give it another chance in the quiet comfort of my own home. To my surprise, not only did it help, but it was incredibly relaxing and enjoyable, as I was able to just sit there in silence for a few minutes and relax. Sure, at first like everyone else I struggled clearing my mind, which can actually be quite frustrating when you are trying so hard to do the opposite. But I think what was more important than anything else for me was the simple action of physically sitting down and deciding I was going to at least try and relax, rather than rushing around trying to cram a few other tasks into the precious spare minutes of the day.

I highly recommend you at least give it a chance and if it's something you are new to or unsure how to do, then there are a variety of apps and videos online you can follow for all levels, abilities and even customisable to the length of your available time.

To start with though, you could try the following:

Relaxing meditating technique

- Either sit in a chair keeping your feet flat on the ground or cross-legged on a comfortable mat or cushion on the floor. Keep your back straight and hands in your lap.

- You need to try and keep fidgeting to a minimum, avoiding sudden movements and impulses. Rather than reaching to scratch an itch, instead try readjusting your body, fighting the urge.

- Close your eyes and focus on your breathing, thinking in your mind 'inhale' and 'exhale' as you take air in through your nose and out through your mouth. Whenever your mind starts to wander, try and go back to simply focusing on your breath. This will help to clear your mind, as you are consciously trying to avoid thoughts.

- After a few minutes when you feel relaxed, try and stop thinking 'inhale' and 'exhale', instead focusing solely on how it feels to breath. Being soothed as you take in and release air out of your system.

- Initially you may find it's hard to maintain focus and it will be common for your mind to wander, especially when first engaging in this practice. If that happens then don't worry about it or let it aggravate you. In those moments simply go back to focusing on your breath, relax and try again.

I know on paper it sounds silly, but remember this is all about personal growth and pushing your comfort zones by trying new experiences and activities.

You can start by engaging in this for as little as five minutes a day, at any time or point you feel like you need to unwind or relax. When you feel comfortable or want to try longer periods, start by increasing it in small increments to 10 or maybe 15 minutes. The aim is for this to become an enjoyable habit. However, if after increasing it too much you begin to have negative feelings towards practicing it (such as boredom), simply reduce the amount of time back to a manageable amount. It helps to partake in this activity at the same time everyday, whether that's first thing in the morning to prepare you for what lies ahead, or late at night when attempting to unwind is up to you.

Meditation definitely takes some getting used to and initially can be frustrating, but just remember this is all part of the process and sticking with it will help improve both your self awareness and control, which can carry over into a range of situations throughout the day.

What if you still can't sleep?

On nights you find yourself still lying in bed, unable to rest, staring at the clock will only make things worse, as you are causing further stress due to the aggravation caused from still being awake. I know what it's like, endlessly tossing and turning, as the more you try to force yourself to fall asleep, the more awake you seem to become. In these circumstances, after a reasonable amount of time (say 20 to 30 minutes), get out of bed and try a relaxing activity such as reading, listening to calming music or meditating. Do it until you feel yourself becoming tired and only then return to bed. Just like with managing stress or reducing anger, sometimes all you need to do is remove yourself from the negative circumstances or environment for a brief period of time. This will aid in reducing stress hormones produced during this time, allowing you to return feeling calmer and more relaxed.

"Don't underestimate the value of doing nothing, of just going along, listening to all the things you can't hear, and not bothering."

- Winnie the Pooh

Final thoughts

That should give you an idea of ways to unwind or relax and a variety of these practices can be incorporated into your routine, regardless of how busy you are. Not only that, but you can adapt them in a way that works for you and hopefully they will open your eyes to other actions you could pursue to help with this part of your development. I really can't stress enough the importance of finding ways to rest and recover. Like I said before, it's all well and good improving your diet and becoming more active, but the only way you will truly achieve balance is by ensuring you take into consideration all the other aspects contributing to your wellbeing.

It's now up to you to think about how you are going to organise your time towards making room for resting. Start with thinking about your evening routine. Are there are any changes you can make to your bedtime ritual? Or if you don't have one then this would be the perfect time to look at establishing one. It doesn't need to be overly fancy or complicated, but simply making some small changes or introducing certain actions can go a long way in helping you relax and unwind. It's all about creating healthy habits and a routine, all while improving the environment in which you rest.

Pillar Four
Diet and nutrition

"Every living cell in your body is made from the food you eat. If you consistently eat junk food then you'll have a junk body."
- Jeanette Jenkins

A healthy diet is a big part of the foundation on which a healthy lifestyle is built and the main aim of this book is to teach and guide you on how to put it all together, without overcomplicating an issue that in essence, should be pretty simple. The goal is to move you away from the mindset of 'dieting', instead aiming to transition you into a way of eating where you never have to diet again. That means no more unachievable restriction, no more counting calories and definitely no more starving yourself, instead replacing those actions with eating healthy nutritious meals, that are not only delicious, but also provide your body with the nutrients it requires to thrive. The reality is that this change in mindset will be the only way to achieve your weight goals, with the added benefit of the results being maintainable long-term. This will lift a huge burden from your day-to-day routine, removing a tremendous amount of unnecessary thought, pressure and obsession. For too long food has taken control of everything from our thoughts to our emotions and our lives. Now that you are reading this, it's finally time to take control for yourself. Before diving into the foundations of nutrition and how to put together a balanced diet, it's important to get a better understanding about your relationships with food, why you eat the way you do, as well as why you have developed your current lifestyle and everyday habits. When you get right down to it, the only way you can focus on actively making changes is by firstly both recognising and acknowledging your behaviours, along with determining how and why they exist.

"If the doctors of today do not become the nutritionists of tomorrow, then the nutritionists of today will become the doctors of tomorrow."
- **The Rockefeller Institute of Medical Research**

The importance of proper nutrition

The ideas surrounding the prominence of proper nutrition are not new and throughout history have been preached by influential figures from around the world. Even as far back as 350 BC its undeniable importance was apparent, as Hippocrates stated 'let food be your medicine and medicine be your food'. If his opinion doesn't sway you enough, then Linus Pauling, a man who had 48 PHDs, won two unshared Nobel prizes, was voted the second most important scientist in the 20th century, and has been described as being to chemistry what Einstein was to physics, claimed that 'by giving the body the right molecules most disease would be eradicated'. That's why nutritional therapy is and should be the medicine of the future and the evidence stacks heavily in favour of stating that many of today's illnesses would not exist, could be prevented, or even reversed if proper nutrition was adopted on a mass scale.

Instead society has become obsessed with treating disease, and this obsession is directly spurring on many of our problems, rather than resolving them. Don't get me wrong, the medical industry has a huge and positive impact on making people's lives better, but too much attention is placed on how to treat illnesses, rather than focusing on preventing them. The easiest way to do this is through the use of proper nutrition, but instead the healthcare system has simply developed into a disease-care system, trying to bandage and quickly discharge a problem, that can't simply just be covered up. If you feel sceptical about that claim, then consider the fact that America has the most advanced medical industry in the world, yet in comparison, it also has the sickest nation. Forty-eight percent of the population are on regular prescription drugs, most commonly for cardiovascular disease and high cholesterol, which surely in itself is enough evidence of the huge problem we have on our hands.

History has shown that the human body is able to fight and recover from severe damage if provided with the right tools to repair itself, and while eating properly doesn't ensure we will remain free from illness, it's the only sure fire way to stack the deck in our favour. So I don't know about you, but for me it makes far more sense to try and unload the gun, rather than trying to dodge a bullet.

When you think about it properly, there really are only three things we can eat – plants, animals or processed foods. The way the human body functions is the result of millions of years of evolution and adapting to gradual changes in environment, and by looking at what our ancestors ate, scientists have been able to establish what kind of nutrients the body has become accustomed to receiving. Since the dawn of mankind people have thrived on a diet of plant based and animal foods, with our intake primarily coming from plant based sources, which were grown, harvested and consumed in their natural form. You might argue that throughout history there have been diseases and famines, however, this in itself is a glaringly obvious history lesson we should be learning from: the diseases and famines have happened as a lack of availability of nutrients, not caused by them! In the modern day most of the plants that were once consumed have been replaced by heavily refined and processed foods, along with the industrialisation of certain processes and ability to mass produce. Through this we have been able to create items that satisfy our palate, seeking pleasure over what we actually need. This hedonistic state has led to people becoming addicted to these products, while at the same time, being starved of essential nutrients.

If you need more convincing, there have been various studies on other cultures that have shown a distinct difference in their rates of diabetes, cancer and heart disease when compared to the Western world, with findings showing that the primary differences come down to diet and nutrition. While these other cultures have a generally lower calorie intake, what they do consume is far higher in nutritional value, made up of a diet consisting largely of wholefoods that undergo little to no processing. This is the direct opposite of our society, where we generally have a high calorie intake that's very low in nutrients and is highly processed using a wide range of ingredients, chemicals and preservatives. When comparing our standards of living with those of less developed countries you would think our risk of these illnesses would surely be lower due to our readily available sources of food and healthcare. But in regards to chronic diseases, the opposite is true. It doesn't take an expert to clearly see how nutrition directly links to the health epidemics we are increasingly facing, and it appears that the significantly lower chance of developing these illnesses in less developed countries is largely due to their limited access to the products we are consuming in high quantities on a daily basis.

The World Cancer Organisation estimates that 'eating five or more servings of fruit or vegetables everyday could prevent 20 percent of all cases of cancer', and this was further supported by an analysis looking at 16 different studies across the US, Europe and Asia. The study involved nearly one million people, and found the average risk of death was reduced by five percent for every portion consumed, maxing out at five portions. That's why five portions is the daily recommendation advertised by the authorities, yet it has been found that 70 percent of people don't even come close to this amount.

The problem is most people don't realise how much of an effect their diet and nutrition has on how they feel and it's only when they start to eat properly and see the benefits from these changes that they realise how much of a negative impact their previous actions were having on their overall wellbeing. That's because food has the power to nourish, heal and make you strong, boosting your mood and energy, all while affecting everything from your happiness to your sleep and mindset. But at the same time, it has the power to leave you with feelings of despair, emptiness, guilt and shame, bringing negativity to everyday life, rather than being a source that enriches it.

So what's the problem?

Part of the issue is that when asked, many people believe they follow moderation, all while being completely oblivious to not only what they are eating, but equally how much. They fail to recognise that while that doughnut on Monday may have been the only doughnut for the week, when combined with the chocolate on Tuesday, pizza on Wednesday and Chinese with a few beers on Friday, they are in fact consuming a wide range of foods that while different in perceived basic form, are all filled with sugar, processed fats, chemicals and empty calories. All of these choices eventually add up, taking a huge toll on both their waistline and health. I'm not saying there's anything wrong with having a doughnut, but the problems start to arise when it's combined with all the other items negatively contributing to a poor diet. Far too many of the food choices people make everyday aren't down to what they need, but rather are merely because of habits, routines and addiction, mostly for momentary satisfaction, regardless of the long-term consequences.

To put it into a more visual perspective, just think about how your car won't run without fuel. And what happens if you put the wrong type of fuel in? It works briefly before breaking down and fails to function properly until you correct the problem, as the fuel you have given it is unable to be processed by the engine in order to make the car move.

Your body functions in very much the same way, which is why if you feel like you are constantly fighting an uphill battle just to make it through the day, low on energy, tired, moody or not your true self, you can guarantee this is largely due to your body lacking the fuel it requires, and the constant physiological wear and tear being placed on it. Without the proper nutrients your body is unable to complete everyday tasks, which is why your health keeps stalling and breaking down, until eventually it gets to the point where it can no longer fight off illness or disease.

With many people I have dealt with, talking about how they truly feel and having an honest reflection on their overall wellbeing, brings about a moment of self-realisation. It's a moment that clicks and makes them realise how much their everyday state of mind is in fact influenced by what they put into their body. It's so obvious when you actually think about it, yet overlooked by the majority of people. But why wouldn't it be overlooked? For so long people have been trapped into feeling this way and it has got to the point where they have simply come to accept that is how they are meant to be feeling. I know that's the reality I was living in for so long, completely unaware of how different things could and should be.

The hardest part of change is all in your head. You need to get over your preconceptions, doubts and stubborn thinking. Once you have, you will start seeing ordinary foods as more appealing, recognising the benefit they have for you, and moving away from the notion that eating healthily is all about bland boring food. This reason is used by many people as a label or excuse to avoid even trying many of these foods, completely unaware of how wrong they actually are. Once your misconceptions clear you will be amazed at how good 'healthy' food can taste and how much more enjoyable life is once you have broken the addiction to sugary, processed foods, and stopped letting them control how you feel.

Throughout this process it's essential to remember that no one is perfect and that we simply can't eat healthily all of the time. In fact, there's absolutely no need to even try. Life's too short to put that much pressure on yourself and by trying to do so all you are doing is setting yourself up for failure. Instead of taking that highly stressful all or nothing approach, in order to achieve and maintain your ideal weight and health, the aim should be to eat healthily most of the time. That way when you do choose to indulge you can do so guilt free, all while doing a minimal amount of harm to your body. This mindset and approach right here is exactly what will be maintainable long term and that is the exact reason why this isn't simply just another diet. This is a way you can eat for the rest of your life, and you can do so knowing that there is no outside force telling you what you can or can't do, and you aren't living a life where your favourite treats are off limits. You will find that adapting to this mindset in itself lifts a huge burden, as that change in thought alone will dramatically change how you think about and see food. Not only that, but it will reduce cravings and increase willpower, thereby having a huge impact on your overall state of mind.

"The best way to capture moments is to pay attention. This is how we cultivate mindfulness. Mindfulness means being awake. It means knowing what you are doing."
- Jon Kabat-Zinn

Mindfulness and learning to listen to your body

An important factor in determining your success in this process will be learning to listen to what your body is telling you and how to recognise the signs of being full. By doing so, you will be able to move away from habits like finishing everything on your plate or constantly indulging, simply because food is there. 'Mindful eating' is a trend that has exploded over the last few years, with ties to everything from Buddhism, to being rooted in Zen or forms of yoga. In principle it's all about reconnecting us with the experience of eating and enjoying our food, all while developing a consciousness about not only what we eat, but also why. For me though, it's far simpler and less spiritual than that, as it's simply about slowing down and taking a moment to enjoy the taste, smell, sound and texture of what you we are eating, trying to enjoy every bite, and stopping when satisfied. It's about recognising physical signs, such as the signals our body sends when we are hungry, and becoming aware of our thoughts and actions, rather than acting on emotions, such as eating for comfort.

Mindfulness in itself is a theme that you will notice coming up throughout this book, but its prominence in regards to the way you eat is more important than ever. It's easy to confuse mindful eating as only being about eating slowly and without being distracted, and while those aspects certainly are important, they are far from the full story. A big part of getting into this mindset is recognising and understanding your relationships with food, why you eat the way that you do and how food makes you feel. Not just emotionally, but physically as well. You need to learn to recognise the triggers that cause you to turn to certain foods, along with finding ways to fulfil your needs that don't revolve around eating. It's all about choosing foods that provide enjoyment on top of nourishment, allowing you to eat for satisfaction and satiety.

Getting this right and under control could very much be a turning point in your life, not just in your weight goals, but in your personal growth and mindset as well. That's why in order to progress, we firstly need to look at the issues involved in more detail.

"Those who think they have no time for healthy eating, will sooner or later have to find time for illness."
- Edward Stanley

Our relationships with food

One of the biggest factors that influences our health is often the most overlooked, and that's our relationship with food. Everyone's relationship with food is different, with how it's used or viewed ranging from fuel to reward, a form of freedom, escape, comfort, or even as punishment. We don't just fall into one category either, as these relationships can fluctuate massively depending on our mood, environment, stress levels, the amount of sleep we get, or any other factors influencing us on the day. For instance, I now recognise that mine can quickly change from fuel to comfort, a shift that has on many occasions taken control of how I behave. Often food is the only thing in life we can control, which is why it's common place for it to unknowingly be used as an outlet to help in times of despair, a coping mechanism that can quickly and easily turn into an addiction. A survey conducted by the American Psychological Association found that in times of stress, one in three people turned to eating as a form of relief, which is evidence in itself that these habits and behaviours need more of our attention. Nevertheless, it's easy to misinterpret that our relationships with food and the habit of over eating are just down to negative circumstances, when in fact, they can just as easily be linked to happiness and positive situations. For instance, social, family gatherings and work events are often based around the concept of eating huge amounts, treating indulgence as a means of celebration, connecting and appreciation.

A huge contributing factor in this issue is the unnecessary pressure that society places on us, as we are constantly led to believe we need to adhere to or achieve stereotypes of the perfect body, that in most cases are simply unobtainable. Yet failing to reach these heights often comes with the connotation that we aren't good enough as people, and this in itself is a huge pressure that further pushes us towards negative behaviours, as questioning our self-worth simply reinforces self-doubt.

People who are obese tend to get the brunt of these negative perceptions, often viewed or labelled as lazy, lacking in willpower or unambitious. But for many it actually revolves around far deeper misunderstood issues, ranging from depression to loneliness, fear, anxiety, stress, or even past traumas or abuse. Studies and interviews with people struggling with obesity have shown the majority want to lose weight and improve their health. From those I have dealt with and spoken to I think it's fair to say that many have even tried every diet imaginable, yet for the majority nothing has worked, and often they simply relapse on any progress they've made. The problem is misperceptions about what it takes causes people to torture themselves following approaches they are led to believe will help, which suggests that the issue at hand is not a lack of desire to do something about it, but is rather down to pursuing the wrong solution. It really is a doubled edged sword, as giving it everything they've got and not seeing results often pushes them deeper into a state of accepting that this is how they were born to be, and further spurs on negative food related behaviours, as a way to try and deal with that acceptance.

We have now reached a point where people who are of a healthy weight are in the minority, with weight gain often being blamed as the cause of many of our health problems. But on the other side of this, what garners little to no attention is the fact that you don't have to be overweight to be sick. Everyone seems to automatically assume that because someone is thin that they are healthy and can eat whatever they want, but the reality is some people just don't store body fat as visibly as others. Medical scans and studies have shown that up to 40 percent of 'thin' people actually have the same metabolic dysfunctions as those who are overweight, meaning that while the physical signs may not be as directly apparent, the long-term implications of their actions are just as severe. Internally thinner-looking people can have a huge build-up of fat and cholesterol, along with being pre-diabetic, having high blood pressure, or a range of other health related issues that are often believed to just be problems for the obese.

These two examples really show how this issue can go from one extreme to another, with people falling at the far side of both ends of the spectrum. For that reason don't assume that just because you perceive someone as eating 'well' all the time that means that he or she has everything figured out. That view point simply adds extra pressure and doubt onto a mindset that's already challenging to overcome. When all is said and done, we are all very different, but one thing many of us have in common is that we are struggling with an internal battle, that's largely brought on by an all or nothing approach and inability to find balance. What's important to take away from this is that everyone has their own relationship with food, and we all struggle from time to time in practicing control, moderation or making the right choices.

It could even be argued that you can look at it from a different perspective, where obesity is now no longer the problem and instead has become the solution to the issues in people's lives. Everyone has instances in their life that has affected them in various ways, from stress to a dysfunctional family situation, abuse, bullying, depression or general unhappiness. The damage caused by these situations varies, with the extent being more long-term in some than others. In response to this we have all established ways in which to try and cope with our emotions, with some people being far more successful at doing so than others. The relationships we have with food are heavily related and connected to our overall mindset and outlook on life, with what we choose to consume often being an expression of how we are feeling. It's because of this that you need to find out what's causing you to behave the way that you do, and actively set about changing your life as a whole. It's normal to have stress and bad days, but it's not normal to live in a situation where you feel like you are so overwhelmed that you are continually spiralling out of control. Life moves so fast and has become so high pressure, that many people simply can't cope, causing their relationships with food and health to suffer. Many studies have led to the conclusion that this is down to the fact that what you eat and how you choose to treat your body are one of the only parts of your life you have complete control over and therefore they are often abused as an outlet for other problems, subconsciously done as an internal power struggle trying to grasp hold of some form of control.

How this has affected me

I remember a time after getting an exam result that didn't go according to plan, where I rushed out and bought a huge cheesecake and tub of chocolate mousse. This was during a period where I had excluded all these 'bad' foods from my diet and was restricting my food intake to be purely what I perceived as healthy 'clean' eating, in an attempt to lose weight. I remember feeling helpless and this resulted in a decision of 'screw it', I'm going to go and get something that will make me feel better (or so I thought). My emotions had taken control of me and that moment pushed me into a state of panic and self-doubt where I ate so much, that I was actually sick afterwards. I was just looking for a feeling of reassurance or comfort that things would be ok. Did it make anything better? No. But at the time of purchasing I genuinely believed that it might. This is a perfect example of a situation where because I had no control over what had happened, I turned to an outlet I could control instead. My mind related the thought of those foods with a feeling of happiness and because I had deprived myself of them for so long, I couldn't stop myself when I finally gave in. Once I started I kept chasing that feeling and started eating merely for the sake of it, just shovelling it away and not actually enjoying or even paying attention to what I was consuming.

But trying to justify that action to myself achieved nothing, as in one way or another life will always be stressful and that's why you can't live tip toeing along until the next thing that pushes you too far. That's why it's essential in these moments you simply stop, take a deep breath, calm down and think it through. I'm sure in most cases that will lead to the realisation that everything will be ok and you don't need to seek out other forms of comfort that may potentially only offer a temporary form of relief. If and when you do face situations like this in the future, going forward you simply need to accept them for what they are, instead of mentally beating yourself up over it. I know that's easier said than done, but what's important now is how you choose to deal with these moments going forward, as nothing in life will ever be perfect and no matter how good things are there will always be moments that challenge and push you towards bad decisions. During moments of high emotions, the body has no connection as to whether or not it's actually hungry and for the majority of comfort eaters, they are simply trying to fill a void that can't be filled with food. If this is the case for you, one of the biggest changes you need to make is to stop eating when you are upset and instead find a new outlet to relieve your emotions.

So ask yourself what would be better to calm yourself down? Maybe go for a walk or run? Listen to some music? Try meditation? Start planning a trip or activity that gives you something to look forward to? Briefly remove yourself from the situation?

Everyone is different, so what works as a release for one person, may not work for another. Just like many things in this process, it will come down to trial and error to find out what's right for you. With all things considered though, it's absolutely essential that you find an outlet to deal with your emotions that has a positive effect on your health. Sure food is the easiest, as it's all around and the most convenient, but more often than not the outlet you are turning to for comfort is only providing momentary relief and in the long run is actually making you feel worse. Not just in your overall health, but also in the moments of guilt and regret that immediately follow, throwing you into a whirlwind of emotions that in turn simply adds insurmountable extra pressure, all of which can potentially push you further into a rut.

"Some rules are nothing but old habits that people are afraid to change."
- Theresa Fowler

Why do you eat the way you do?

Your relationships with food heavily influences the dietary decisions you make and this can either help you thrive, or put a huge strain on your overall health. Matters are made even worse when you continue to repeatedly make the same bad decisions day after day, which as we saw in the habits section, is an easy routine to fall into and get stuck in. This is especially true when it comes to poor daily food choices, which is why in order to successfully rectify the problem, you firstly need to understand its causes, as this awareness will in turn allow you to actively focus on changing your behaviours. Improving your relationships with food will in large come down to forming new habits, along with changing the way you eat so that it's primarily based around healthy nutritious foods and in some cases even changing the environments in which your meals are consumed. That's the only way to break the addiction, which is why it's essential that you recognise that there is in fact a problem to begin with. It's important to remember that everyone is different, and while one person may turn to salt, another may turn to fat or sugar, and because of that, the answer to improving our eating habits can't be pigeonholed into a one size fits all solution. But what can be done is to find the basis for your decisions and from there, find ways in which to change them. This will allow us to actively take steps towards improving your relationships with food, and will come hand in hand with adapting to a new way of eating, free from restriction, in addition to improving your overall mindset and outlook on life.

The perception you have of food can heavily influence the way in which you use it, which is why food manufactures spend millions on product development in order to get the perfect balance between texture, smell, fizz and crunch. This is often done with complete disregard for how much sugar, fat or salt it requires, and because of this they are able to develop highly satisfying products, that create sensations you relate to certain foods and thoughts, exciting your brain and keeping you wanting more. Many of these foods have little to no nutritional value, all while being extremely high in calories. This means that even when consumed in large amounts, your stomach sends signals to your brain saying that you are still hungry, causing you to continue to overeat. That's why it's so easy to finish that entire pack of cookies, or get through that entire bag of potato chips, and still be left wanting more.

The extent that manufacturers go to when creating their products doesn't stop there though, as the whole process dives far deeper on a biological level of how the body responds than you would ever have imagined. Meaning it's not merely just a situation of combining certain flavours until they taste good. Your brain is designed to like variety, which is why if you regularly eat the same meal over and over you get bored. That's why 'junk' foods are designed in a way that avoids those sensory responses, giving you a sufficient amount of taste to keep you interested, without stimulating your brain enough to get bored of them. This causes you to eat more while feeling less satisfied, and heavily contributes towards manipulating you into getting addicted.

This is done through the sugars and fats in these foods triggering receptors in your brain, momentarily boosting your levels of the feel good hormone serotonin, which makes you want to keep eating. Your brain registers these feelings and causes it to trigger the sensation of you having that happiness again the next time you see, smell or even hear about that food, even causing you to salivate over the thought of it and producing the cravings you feel over certain products.

The relationship implanted in your mind between foods and emotions is what causes the desire for you to turn to them when feeling a certain way. This explains the perceived belief that a particular food can make you feel better in a negative situation, thereby causing you to crave it again the next time you feel that way. This in turn develops a habit of how you respond when facing these emotions, and often these thoughts can be related to our childhood, where we relate certain foods and emotions to feelings of safety and comfort.

This addiction is similar to what drug addicts and alcoholics go through, with their brain sending signals to the body that it needs that substance, genuinely believing in the blink of an eye it could make everything better. Often these emotions can cause huge urges, withdraw symptoms and mental aggravation, leading to a huge internal battle that can be extremely difficult not to give into.

Your relationships with food say a lot about how you view yourself and it has been proven that body dissatisfaction is the number one cause of food restriction. These negative thoughts can make you desperate for that feeling of comfort, which can force you into a continual battle with self-acceptance, where you never feel good enough. This aggravating mindset can cause these feelings and emotions to continue to manifest when people reach their goals, as still in their mind they are striving to reach a level of perfection that's simply unobtainable. This is because while they may have achieved what they believed they initially wanted, during this process they failed to tackle the root of the problem, which at the very foundation remains their relationships with food and the way they eat. Simply losing the weight didn't change that and in many ways can leave them no better off mentally than they were before. So while they may look great, internally their struggle might be worse than before, as their entire journey has been a miserable endeavour, based all around restriction. This is why for many, any progress is quickly lost or undone.

People tend to approach trying to get slimmer with starvation tactics and they do so by convincing themselves that it's for the good of their health, obsessing over weight loss and making themselves miserable. In turn all this does is place a further strain on how they view food, creating an association where certain foods are seen as forbidden if they want the body they desire. This is why for the majority of people I'm so against diets based heavily on restriction, as in many cases they do far more harm than good. The case that stands out the most in this regard was that of a lady who was training for an athletic event and became obsessed with 'clean' eating and counting every calorie she consumed. This mindset placed an unbelievable amount of extra pressure on her already negative relationships with food, causing a huge amount of misery, where she constantly relapsed and binged, which would send her into a meltdown mentally, panicking it would mess up her training and ruin her career. This really wasn't a healthy way to live and it was only after she changed her behaviours that she realised how much less she craved certain items and when she did, she could happily consume them without any feelings of guilt or despair, and actually enjoy them for what they were. Another take away point from this case is that negative relationships with food don't just affect people who are obese, and it's an issue that can impact anyone from office workers to professional athletes.

Exercise and relationships with food

Enter any gym and you will often find people addicted to exercise, spending hours everyday on a treadmill trying to lose weight, yet staying the same in terms of their progress, until they either get frustrated with their results or burn themselves out. Don't get me wrong, exercise is an amazing activity, with so many health benefits and as you have already seen I'm a huge proponent of everyone in one way or another becoming more active. But the honest truth is that no matter how hard you try, you simply can't exercise your way out of a bad diet and even trying to do so can play a huge role in influencing your relationships with food.

An example of how truly important this is can be seen in the Journal of Obesity, who conducted one of the most rigorous studies on physical activity and weight loss ever done. They took 200 overweight, sedentary adults, placed them on an aggressive exercise routine and told them to leave their diets unchanged. From this they were able to fully understand the effects gained solely through exercise over an extended period of time.

Over the course of the year, participants were monitored to ensure they were exercising at the studies required rate of five to six hours a week (more than double the government recommendation of two and a half hours a week). The findings will undoubtedly come as a huge shock, as at the end of the study the men had lost an average of 3.5 pounds and the women around 2.5 pounds, leaving almost all participants still overweight or obese. Dr. Anne McTiernan, the lead author of the study concluded that while "adding exercise to a diet program helps, for weight loss you are going to get much more impact with diet changes."

This study gives us a good idea about why so many people give up on the idea of exercising when they realise that simply moving more isn't a miracle cure to their weight problems, as it doesn't give them free reign to neglect the other areas needed to see results, such as their diet, mindset and recovery. Yet that's the approach far too many take.

While everyone burns different amounts of calories during activities based on their individual attributes, to put it all in perspective, below are some ball park figures produced by studies on how long it takes to burn off certain foods:

1) One can of coke would require a 55-minute walk
2) One Cookie a 20-minute jog
3) One Slice of pizza a 30-minute bike ride
4) A 52-minute run for a small chocolate bar

That means for your average 160-pound/73kg person, an hour of running burns around 600 calories, weightlifting burns around 365 calories and cycling around 290 calories. When compared to a sugary doughnut containing 350 calories, you can clearly see we simply don't have the time or energy to balance it all out through exercise alone.

This is made even worse by the fact that when we are asked how many calories we think they burnt during exercise, our estimations tend to be way off, regularly thinking we have burnt double, if not more than what we actually have. This may not sound like much of a problem, but it is when this belief is used to justify our food choices after a workout, often causing us to eat more calories than we otherwise would have and far more than our activity burnt off. That right there is the direct reason why so many people are so mystified when they are doing everything they can to move more, yet still aren't seeing any weight loss, as they completely disregard their behaviours, in most cases not even realising they are doing so. Subconsciously it's easy to turn to food as a reward, unknowingly justifying it to yourself due to the internal belief that a positive action cancels out a negative one, without realising how counterproductive this may be.

"The secret of change is to focus all of your energy, not on fighting the old,
but on building the new."
- Socrates

What now?

Orlando Health conducted a survey of over 1000 people to try and better understand the general view on what it takes to lose weight. Unsurprisingly, 31 percent of those asked believed exercise was the biggest barrier, with 26 percent thinking it's what they ate. Only ten percent of those questioned recognised the psychological factors involved and this may indicate why so many people struggle with not only losing weight, but also keeping it off long-term. That's why If you truly want to progress in not only this process, but also improving your overall health, you need to shift your focus onto what's actually important, like your health, happiness and wellbeing. I know it's hard, especially having to break all the pre-beliefs and perceptions that have been programmed into you throughout your entire life in regards to not only what it takes to lose weight, but also how food is viewed or treated.

I have worked with many people who couldn't believe the change in how they behaved and viewed foods when they finally stopped dieting and started to eat for both health and pleasure instead, as by improving both your lifestyle and relationship with food, you will see healthy weight loss as a lasting by-product of these changes. Not only that, but you will be able to keep it off, an accomplishment very few others seem to be able to achieve.

The reality is highly restrictive diets simply don't work, as from a psychological point of view, the more you tell yourself you can't have something, the more you become fixated on it, craving it until the eventual snapping and binging. If you are anything like me, then I'm sure you can think of countless occasions when on a diet you have told yourself you will just have one cookie, piece of chocolate or bowl of ice cream, only to land up finishing the entire pack or tub. This is down to your mind obsessing over what you have mentally restricted to the point that it can't take anymore, and when you give in saying you will only have a small amount, you instead land up binging, unable to stop. Queue the feelings of guilt and self-doubt, followed by giving up and quitting the diet all together.

The worst part is that deep down, most of us know that dieting doesn't work, yet we do it anyway, as we believe that's what needs to be done in order to lose weight. At least when it's over we can say we tried to change, and can go right back to the way things were, using this brief ordeal of punishment as justification to continue making bad decisions, until our actions guilt us into repeating the process again.

That's why if you truly want to change and improve this part of your wellbeing for the better, then you need to stop hiding, sit down and honestly ask yourself where in life you aren't satisfied, along with what's directly causing all of these problems and triggering you to behave how you do. Chances are it's playing a huge role in pushing you towards eating the way that you do and this is no doubt having a huge impact on your overall mental, physical and emotional health. It's only by doing this that you'll be able to embrace and face the problem head on.

As hard as it may be to admit these things to yourself, it's unfortunately a part of your journey that you need to deal with.

- Is it too much pressure at home or work?
- Old traumas still affecting you?
- A negative social or work environment?
- Being surrounding by constant temptation?
- Feeling like you are lost and alone?
- Not being happy with where you are and no clue where you are going?

The cause will be different for everyone and may be along completely different lines to the examples given and it is likely it may even be a combination of more than one factor. It's essential though that you are honest with yourself about not only what's causing you problems, but also how you have been dealing with them so far.

Once you recognise how and why you behave the way that you do, it will be up to you to actively ensure that you make a conscious effort to change how you respond. That's why I want you to thoroughly think about instances where you have reacted in a way you would like to change or avoid, along with a different response you would rather make in the future. This could be anything from going for a walk to listening to music, or any of the others mentioned previously in this section. Just ensure that whatever you choose as your form of release has nothing to do food, or other destructive substances.

The reason why I want you to do this is because it will enable you to recognise the next time you are placed in this situation and reacting this way. This will allow you to mentally focus and practice how you would like to respond instead. Then regardless of how hard it is, as and when you encounter the situation you need to ensure you respond accordingly with the new action you have set yourself up to take. When done enough times, that response will be the new habit you have formed. I know it's tough, but it will get easier every time that you do it.

Other ways to improve your relationships with food

After a long day there are very few things more relaxing then putting our feet up in front of the TV and turning on anything that will get our minds off the stresses we faced that day. But one of the major problems with eating while watching TV or when distracted is that our focus is on something entirely different, and not what we are consuming. This is a huge issue, as one review on the matter considered the results found in 24 studies and determined that distractions during a meal led to consuming around ten percent more calories in that sitting. This can add up to a substantial amount of excess food, especially if done every day. Not only that, but it has been found that when you are not focused on your meal you get less enjoyment from it, which in itself spurs on negative behaviours. This gets worse when you consider that eating in this manner can also cause us to forget what we have eaten, which is often why an hour after dinner you head straight to the snack cupboard after seeing a commercial for your favourite treat on TV. Acting out of instinct, with complete disregard for what you are actually doing.

That's why one of the easiest ways to start developing a healthier relationship with food is to start eating at a table, where you can apply your full attention to your actions and what you are doing. You could use this time to gather your thoughts, emotions, reflect on your day, and this is also a great way to connect the family. It teaches kids as well as ourselves to savour and appreciate what is being eaten, rather than relating meal times to sitting in front of a TV eating huge quantities, where the eating experience is often rushed with little regard for what's being consumed.

If these are changes you want to pursue, then one approach you could take is to ensure that on Monday to Thursday evenings you eat at a table away from the TV, then allow yourself to be more lenient and relaxed on the weekend.

Aside from changing the environment in which meals are consumed, another approach is to start preparing your own meals, and you can do so by learning to cook healthy and nutritious meals. I know many people view cooking as hard, a hassle, something they don't know how to do or simply don't have time for. But trust me, it's a highly rewarding and engaging experience, that everyone could benefit from adding more of into their lives.

Not only does cooking give you control over what goes into your body, but it teaches you to appreciate food, enabling you look at it as more than simply fuel, and learn to value it for what it is. There are so many incredible flavours and cuisines out there, many of which we often completely disregarded in favour of the same old regular fast food options. Learning to cook is far easier and less time consuming than most people think and there's no need to over complicate it. Cooking also gives you a further outlet to relax, and provides you with a platform for your creative side to take control. You just need to remember it's not about making fancy gourmet meals, but rather all about using fresh ingredients and making meals that you enjoy. These days I very rarely look at or even consider recipes, instead opting to build dishes around ingredients and flavours I have learned over the years go together. This complete freedom when you create a delicious meal is highly rewarding and one of the few aspects in life where you can simply go with how you feel. Although that's my preferred approach, on the other side of this countless people love opening cookbooks and using them for ideas and inspiration of what to try next. There's no right or wrong approach, all that matters is giving it a go and finding out what works best for you. After a long day it may even be exactly what you need to unwind.

I know many people turn to convenience in the evening when they are tired, but personally I find cooking an extremely relaxing activity that really helps with relieving stress after a long day. I put this down to the fact it's an action that I can engage in that's completely different from anything else I have done that day, thereby helping me switch off from work and focus on something else.

Final thoughts

From reading this section hopefully you will have reassessed your views and opinions on the approaches you have taken in the past to achieve your weight goals, as well as evaluated your thoughts and behaviours in regards to how you use, treat and view food. The mistake most people make is focusing too much on the physical elements of weight loss - over exercising and undereating, as that's what society has told them they need to do in order to shed those excess pounds. However, where they are going wrong is overlooking the emotional aspects that are involved within the process.

The reality is that every time you make a decision on what to eat you are choosing what's most important to you in that moment. Is it health and nourishment? Or satisfaction and indulgence? That's not to say that healthy foods can't be delicious and satisfying. But for arguments sake to simplify and illustrate this point I'm going to separate them.

Personally on a day-to-day basis I get the majority of my food from clean, unprocessed, wholefood sources, as I'm eating for health and nourishment. Because of that, most of what I eat revolves around a wide range of fruits and vegetables, lean cuts of meat, complex carbohydrates and healthy fats. I have however learned to prepare them in a way that's delicious, so it really is a win-win situation. Sure initially (and some nights) it takes some extra effort, but if you weigh up the pros and cons, it's a clear winner, for me anyway. Then at times when I'm eating with family or friends, enjoying a social environment or relaxing, I'll eat for indulgence. By approaching the way I eat in this manner,

I don't have to think twice about having that burger, pizza or cheesecake. Best of all, I can do so guilt free and enjoy it for what it is. You will find that by having these products less often you enjoy them more, as in many ways they lose their appeal or satisfaction when consumed each and every day. Changing the way that I eat and approach food has had the knock on effect of improving my relationships with food, which in turn has made me mentally stronger, and in most cases it no longer takes control of how I behave.

In the introduction to this book I said I would be helping you take taking a different approach and hopefully now you are starting to see why. That's why there will be no more strict, inflexible and rigid plans punishing yourself every day. No more feeling like a failure because you chose to eat something you enjoy and definitely no more starving yourself nutritionally and emotionally. The illusion with dieting is that it's achievable and the realisation that people who embark on them are destined to fail from the start can be massively freeing for not only your mindset, but also the way in which you can approach food in the future.

Rather than following a set of rules and guidelines, instead I want you to shatter the glass ceiling that is the norm and apply your focus to listening to your body and recognising what it needs, not creating a separation where you make yourself miserable only eating what you are told you have to. That's why this book involves no special tricks or gimmicks, there's no magic pill or secret formula. It's all about making sustainable healthy lifestyle changes to improve your health. That's not saying it will be easy to adapt to and it definitely isn't giving you free reign to devour everything in sight. But what it is saying is that you can occasionally indulge without all the negative emotions that follow. So no weight loss won't happen overnight, but it will be lasting, enjoyable and maintainable.

The basics of nutrition

"He who takes medicine and neglects diet wastes the skill of his doctors."
- Chinese Proverb

Eating for health is about more than just reducing your intake of highly refined, processed, fatty or sugary products and in many ways, consuming the right foods is just as, if not more important than avoiding the wrong ones. In order to properly function your body needs a range of both macro and micronutrients to effectively perform everyday tasks, as they are essential for everything from growth to repair or fighting disease. I'll warn you now: this section could easily be turned into an entire book, so you will probably be pleased to hear I have condensed it down to only covering what you need to know. The following pages will cover the basics of nutrition, which will be followed by what ingredients to use, and how to structure it all in a maintainable way that works for you.

So what actually is 'food'?

Foods can be broken into two main categories:

Macronutrients; which are protein, carbohydrates and fat.

Micronutrients; which are vitamins and minerals.

In most cases you get these from a variety of foods and it's pretty common for foods to comprise of a range of different nutrients. For instance, some vegetables are high in micronutrients, carbohydrates and contain some protein, whereas meat is higher in protein and micronutrients, while often being lower in carbohydrates.

In addition, I have included water and fibre into this section, as sufficient intake of both is essential for your wellbeing.

Macronutrients

Protein

Protein is made up of amino acids (organic compounds which bond together in long chains), which are used in the creation of everything from tissues such as muscle, skin, organs and tendons, to other molecules including enzymes, hormones and various chemicals in your brain. In essence they are the building blocks of your body, as they are vital for health and everyday functions such as growth and repair. The risks associated with protein deficiency range from increased injuries, to a lack of energy, trouble sleeping, thinning of hair, depression, edema (swelling) and a loss of muscle. There are a total of 20 amino acids you require, 11 of which can be produced by your body, meaning you need to get the other nine from the foods you consume. Animal protein contains all of these essential amino acids, which is why they are most commonly referred to as a 'complete' protein source. Plant based sources on the other hand are described as 'incomplete', as most don't contain the complete range. It's because of this that people with a vegetarian or vegan diet tend to be far more likely to have a protein deficiency, however this is completely avoidable with some careful planning, selection, or even potentially supplementing.

The amount of protein required varies from person to person and is largely dependent on their lifestyle, activity levels and body composition. But with that being said, the average person needs protein to constitute to around 15 percent of their total intake, which is around 50 to 60 grams per day. This does however fluctuate massively depending on individual circumstances, as people involved in regular exercise, manual jobs, pregnant women, or recovering from surgery will be breaking down muscle at a much higher rate, and because of that they will require substantially higher amounts of protein to support with recovery or repair. In some cases, benefit can be seen from as much as 45 percent of calories coming from protein, however that's very much the top end of the scale and 25 to 35 percent is generally a more reasonable amount for those who fall into this category.

There seems to be a reoccurring myth that a high protein diet can damage your kidneys, but evidence has repeatedly refuted this claim. In fact, it has actually been found that for your average healthy person a diet that's higher in protein is actually beneficial for health. Research has shown that eating more protein not only keeps you feeling fuller for longer, but it also burns more calories, therefore making it a much overlooked tool in weight loss. Higher intake also helps preserve muscle mass, which is essential when trying to drop those extra pounds. That's because the process of losing weight requires that you place yourself in a calorie deficit, and therefore often results in a combination of both fat and muscle loss. This is exactly what you don't want, and why low calorie restrictive diets can actually do far more harm than good. A loss of too much muscle mass can drastically slow down your metabolism, as well as bringing about a whole host of other negative effects on your health.

That's why overall I am a huge proponent for the majority of people adapting to a diet that's higher in protein, based largely around lean cuts of meat and other high quality sources such as fish, eggs, dairy, beans and legumes. This becomes increasingly more important as you age, as you become unable to use protein as efficiently. That means you need sufficiently larger amounts to prevent the health risks associated with sarcopenia (loss of muscle mass associated with aging) and osteoporosis.

Please note

Don't get too caught up in stressing over what percentage of your intake is coming from any one source, as there certainly is no need for you to start measuring or mapping everything out. I'm just telling you the rough amounts needed so that you have a general understanding of what's required, and later on we will look at how to determine portion sizes without counting calories.

Carbohydrates

Carbohydrates play a big role in a healthy diet, as they are essential for supporting everyday functions and providing readily available energy. They come in a variety of shapes, forms and sizes, from bread to pasta or oats, but in essence they can be broken down into three categories:

Monosaccharides: which is the more technical term for sugars that are commonly known as simple carbohydrates. The name is given due to their chemical structure, as they are made up of a single cell. Monosaccharides include glucose, fructose and galactose. Glucose is the sugar produced when your body breaks down carbohydrates that you eat, which is why it's commonly known as blood sugar. So whenever you hear someone talk about blood sugar levels, what they are referring to is the amount of glucose in the blood. Fructose on the other hand is the sugar found naturally in fruit and processed products in the form of sucrose, and galactose is the sugar found in dairy. Your liver converts both of these into glucose, before then releasing them into the blood for use.

Disaccarides: are two monosaccharides joined together and include sucrose (commonly table sugar) and lactose (the sugar found in milk).

Polysaccharides: are composed of many sugar molecules linked together and tend to be associated with complex carbohydrates (such as wheat, oats and vegetables).

You are probably thinking that sounds like a load of overly complicated science babble that by the end of this page you will no doubt have forgotten about. In fact, you may even be thinking what was the second one again? Disaccarwhat? And you are right, for the most part it is, as it's not something you overly need to know. However, what is important is to understand is that regardless of the source, all carbohydrates are all broken down by the body into glucose/sugar molecules, with the main difference being the rate at which this is done. The reason why this is so important is that this rate dictates the influence they have on your body, and the easiest way to determine and understand this further is through use of what's known as the Glycemic Index (GI).

The Glycemic Index

The Glycemic Index is basically a ranking system used as a measurement out of 100 to describe how quickly different carbohydrates raise blood sugar levels. Each carbohydrate-based food is assigned a number depending on its influence, with anything under 55 being consider low, 56 to 69 medium and 70+ as high. The GI of a food influences everything from how quickly energy is released to energy levels, how fat is stored and the impact it has on blood sugar levels.

To put this into perspective:

Your body can't directly distinguish between a chocolate bar and some broccoli (yes, when it's broken down it becomes sugar as well) as they are digested the same way, but since the chocolate bar is metabolised at a much faster rate, it therefore rapidly spikes insulin levels. The broccoli on the other hand takes longer to be broken down, allowing levels to remain stable.

Why is this so important?

Constantly changing blood sugar levels can have a huge influence on your health, playing a direct role in the development of chronic diseases such as diabetes, and is a huge contributor towards issues such as obesity. What's more, it can lead to fluctuating energy levels, problems maintaining focus, changes in mood, headaches, along with being directly linked to over eating and cravings. These are just a few of the issues at hand, which is why it's absolutely essential you try to find ways to keep your levels as stable as possible. The easiest way to do this is to stick to primarily low GI wholefoods, such as vegetables and complex carbohydrates.

However, one factor people often overlook when considering the GI of a food is what else it's consumed with. You see, when you combine high GI foods with low GI ones, it decreases the overall GI of the meal. Therefore, combining various sources averages it out and reduces the overall impact higher GI foods have on how you feel. That's why personally if I know I'm going to be indulging in something sweet or high in sugar, wherever possible I try to do so after firstly having a nutritious low GI meal, made up primarily of starchy carbohydrates such as brown rice or whole wheat pasta, and vegetables. This drastically decreases the impact it has on my blood sugar levels, and reduces the overall damage that could potentially have been caused.

Anything else?

One final myth I would like to clear up is the idea that eating carbohydrates after a certain time makes you fat. It's a common belief that if you eat carbohydrates after six in the evening, then your body will be unable to properly respond to the change in insulin levels, thereby making it more likely that they will be stored as body fat and cause weight gain. This is simply just another situation where a misconception that sounds like it could be true is accepted as fact, with no scientific backing to support it. Research conclusively proves this couldn't be farther from the truth, as the reality is excess calories are what cause weight gain, regardless of where they come from or the time of day they are consumed. As long as you are eating healthy balanced meals and not going overboard with any one nutrient, then you really don't need to overthink any other aspects involved.

Fats

Sufficient intake of healthy fats is vital for improving your wellbeing. In fact, from a health perspective, one of the best things you can do is stop fearing consuming fats and instead ensure sufficient amounts are incorporated into your diet. Fats are required for a range of everyday functions, from protecting organs to regulating hormone levels, providing insulation and acting as a source of energy. Not only that, but they are essential for the absorption of vitamins A, D, E and K, meaning that without sufficient fat intake your body is unable to properly absorb these vitamins. Therefore, even if you are eating a most healthy diet, filled with fruit and vegetables, many of the nutrients consumed could be wasted and not put to use. This in turn leads to deficiencies, even if you are consuming adequate amounts. Dietary fat aids in stabilising your blood sugar levels and is highly satiating, helping to keep you full, along with curbing hunger and cravings - all factors that are vital when trying to keep weight loss or maintenance on track, in addition to improving your relationships with food.

The fats you consume can be split into various different forms and without getting too technical in the chemistry behind it all, they are categorised according to the way in which carbon atoms are bonded within the chain. The main types are saturated fats, which are made of single bonds, and unsaturated fats, which have one or more double bonds.

Saturated fats tend to be solid at room temperature and primarily come from animal products such as: butter, cheese, meat, coconut oil and milk.

Unsaturated fats on the other hand are liquid at room temperature and come in two forms:

Monounsaturated fats: found primarily in avocados, olive oil and nuts.

Polyunsaturated fats: found in seeds, fish, sunflower oil, nuts and in small amounts in leafy greens.

You have no doubt heard of the "healthy vs unhealthy fats" issue, and regardless of their molecular bonds, you can in fact classify them based on how they affect our health. Healthy fats from wholefood sources that are essential for everyday health can be placed on one side, with highly processed variations that are linked to obesity and disease on the other. Ideally you want a diet filled with an array of healthy fats, with the best sources to turn to including; extra virgin olive oil, avocados, coconut oil, seeds and nuts.

On the other side of this, you want to consume a minimal amount of processed oils and trans fats. Processed and fast foods tend to primarily contain what is known as hydrogenated fat. These are a man-made form of polyunsaturated fat and are largely linked to the majority of the health risks discussed thus far.

The myth about saturated fat

For decades misperceptions have led people to believe that saturated fats are the direct cause of heart disease and high levels of cholesterol, but new research has concluded that this is far from the case. The reason for the change in opinion is that these health problems are actually relatively new, whereas the human race has been consuming saturated fats since the beginning of their existence. You simply can't blame something we have been eating for thousands of years with no issues for the epidemics we are currently facing, which suggests that saturated fats have merely been used as a scape goat to cover up the fact that these health problems began during the inception of highly refined, processed sugary foods. Therefore, making saturated fat far from the dangerous villain it has been portrayed to be.

Nevertheless, while that means you can be less concerned about the risks associated with the consumption of saturated fats, there still isn't enough evidence supporting what the optimal daily intake amount should be, and the United States Department of Agriculture still recommends keeping intake levels to less than ten percent of your daily calorie intake. However, it's important to note that percentage is based on flawed research, dating back to when saturated fats were still believed to be linked to heart disease. In all likelihood these guidelines will be revised in the near future, once more research is conducted and there's a clearer indication of what we should actually be doing. But just to be on the safe side, until more is known on the issue my advice is that you aim to get most of your fat intake from unsaturated sources wherever possible. Be that as it may, there's an abundance of research preaching the health benefits of coconut oil, which is a saturated fat. This in itself suggests evidence in a changing of the tides and opinions, but as with everything else, a balance of everything is key.

Micronutrients

Vitamins and minerals

Briefly scan pretty much any isle or shelf in your local supermarket and everywhere you look will be products claiming to have added vitamins and minerals. The sad thing is though that many of these products are simply using a clever marketing ploy to package a processed product as something healthy, when chances are it actually has no health boosting properties at all. While it's not the case for all of them, many of these products make promises that in reality are far too good to be true and are simply playing up to the latest trends, catering to what consumers have been led to believe they need. Nevertheless, while these tactics are often misleading or a scam, the benefits and necessity for adequate intake of micronutrients is very real, and it's an area of health that far too many people are neglecting.

Your body needs micronutrients in varying amounts, as they are required to perform millions of physiological processes and functions throughout your body everyday. While they have no calorific value, just a few of their responsibilities include acting as antioxidants and manufacturing antibodies to boost your immune system to fight off disease, balancing hormones, producing energy, building cells, regulating metabolism, protecting arteries, making healthy skin, in addition to being vital for your brain and nervous system. So as you can see, they are vital for pretty much every function related to your health and wellbeing.

At first glance it's easy to get confused between vitamins and minerals, due to the fact that they are both classified as micronutrients and have the same basic premise. However, they do differ in their basic chemical forms.

Vitamins are known as organic compounds, as they are vulnerable to and can be broken down by air, heat, light or time. That means that nutrients can be lost during picking, transporting, processing, preparing, storage and even cooking.

Minerals on the other hand are inorganic elements. They are far more stable and hold their chemical structure in most circumstances they may be exposed to. Think of them as being some of the most basic structures on earth, like the elements in the Periodic Table. They are either close combinations of the elements such as salt - $NaCl$, or standalone molecules such as iron - Ir. While they remain undamaged in cooking, they can however still be lost in water when boiling.

The other major difference between the two is that while all vitamins are essential and required by your body, only some minerals are deemed as essential.

Vitamins

Vitamins can be separated into two distinct categories:

Fat-soluble: consisting of vitamin A, D, E and K.

These are found primarily in fatty foods and animal products such as milk, dairy, eggs, vegetable oils, oily fish and butter.

Although your body needs to use these nutrients to properly function on a daily basis, you don't need to consume them everyday. This is because when consumed, your body stores excess amounts in your fat tissues and liver for future use. Excessive intake can in some cases be harmful, however with a balanced diet this is unlikely to be an issue for concern.

Water-soluble: consisting of Vitamin C, B vitamins and folic acid.

These are found in a variety of foods, including vegetables, fruits, milk, dairy, grains and potatoes. These nutrients aren't stored in your body and therefore are required more frequently, as excess amounts are excreted when more than is needed is consumed. Excessive intake is generally not harmful and you should be aiming to consume foods containing these nutrients everyday.

Minerals

Minerals originate in rocks and metal ores, so therefore are present in soil. That means they are primarily consumed by eating either plants or animals that have eaten plants and to some extent from drinking water. Just like fat-soluble vitamins, your body is able to store minerals for future use if intake becomes low. One of the main problems with processed foods is that minerals are lost during their creation. For instance, when whole grains are refined, potassium, chromium and iron are removed. That's why it's important you make the switch to unrefined sources wherever possible, as if you don't, then you are potentially excluding a whole range of nutrients from your diet.

Where do you get them from?

You primarily get vitamins and minerals in minute quantities from the foods that you consume. There are however some exceptions, including vitamin D, which is made by the skin with the use of natural sunlight, and vitamin K and biotin which are produced by your intestines. It's becoming increasingly common for people to use supplements to boost their intake and while this is better than nothing, you should be aiming to get as many nutrients as possible from actual food sources. This is in most cases easily achievable with a bit of thought and planning, without any inconvenience or having to overthink it.

"The food you eat can be either the safest and most powerful form of medicine or the slowest form of poison."

- Ann Wigmore

Deficiencies

Studies have irrefutably shown that a diet rich in both vitamins and minerals can be directly related to preventing, fighting, treating and even reversing diseases, whereas a diet filled with deficiencies can lead to a whole host of health problems and development of chronic illnesses. The problem at hand is imbalances, as when your body is not provided with what it needs, various processes shut down and it is unable to properly function, due to not being given the right tools to optimally perform. In fact, research is continually starting to support the ideas of Dr. Bruce Ames, who in 2006 presented an award winning idea called the 'Triage Theory', which sheds some further light on this notion. This theory dictates that when the human body isn't being supplied with the nutrients it requires, it diverts what little resources it does get towards supporting essential functions for short-term survival, at the expense of the processes vital for long-term health. For instance, it may prioritise supporting heart function over DNA repair, as that's the more immediate risk to the body's wellbeing. Triage Theory states that micronutrient deficiencies impact your long-term health, and in turn promote age related diseases.

With Western cultures largely processed diets, it can accurately be speculated that a considerable amount of people are potentially deficient in a range of micronutrients and this is affecting their health in a variety of ways. Whether that's long-term damage such as cancer, diabetes, heart disease, dementia or arthritis, or more short term effects such as low energy, mood, stress, focus or overall happiness, will be down to a case by case basis.

How do you know if you have a deficiency?

The only way you can truly tell if you are deficient in certain vitamins and minerals is through blood tests and other examinations such as tests on strands of hair. But these can often be costly and inconvenient procedures, with huge debates over their accuracy. There are however certain signs you can look for depending on how you are feeling. The easiest way to avoid them is to ensure you get the full range by eating a diet based around nutrient dense foods, coming primarily from a wide range of wholefood sources. This is important to take into consideration, as while one food may be high in certain nutrients, it will be lacking in others, as no single food contains a sufficient amount of all of your daily requirements. For instance, fruits and vegetables contain a substantial amount of vitamin C, whereas Vitamin B12 is found primarily in meat, dairy and seafood. This is why it's essential you have a balanced and varied diet, free from exclusions or restrictions.

One wide misconception I would like to point out about deficiencies is that they are just found in individuals with a diet consisting of largely processed foods. While obviously they might be at a higher risk, the reality is that people who eat 'clean' are under substantial threat as well. This is because the concept of clean eating often causes people to have a highly restricted diet, tending to mostly consume the same foods day in and day out. This small amount of variety limits exposure to the nutrients required for sustainable health, as there's not enough variance to cover everything they need. This is why the perceived healthy diet of bland chicken, broccoli and rice consumed by many athletes is in fact highly detrimental to their health. Thus while it may work for short term performance or developing the aesthetic look they desire, from a health perspective it can be extremely damaging.

Most common deficiencies

Due to the amount of vitamins and minerals, all with varying functions I think going into too much detail on every nutrient will simply just over complicate matters. There's simply far too much too take in and it's unnecessary for the average person to know all of it. Especially since while it's possible to be deficient in almost any nutrient, some are highly unlikely, regardless of your diet.

So rather than turning the remainder of this section into a painfully dull science lesson, going through every vitamin and mineral one by one, I have decided instead to just focus on the most common deficiencies and how to avoid them.

My advice is to see if what you are currently eat contains any of the foods listed and if not, then ensuring you find ways to incorporate or increase their intake into your diet.

Vitamin D – if you work in an office, spend most of your days indoors, or live in a country that fails to get regular sunshine, then chances are you are deficient in Vitamin D. It's essential in almost every cell in your body, with symptoms ranging from fatigue to muscle ache and tiredness, with long term deficiency potentially leading to an increased risk of fractures caused by bone loss. It's an understatement to say that if you want to improve how you feel, then you need to increase your intake. I regularly encounter people who are severely deficient, with clear signs being that they are exhausted, moody, depressed, have a lack of energy, feel stuck in a rut and generally overwhelmed and down on life. If you can't or unable to find ways to get more sunshine, then ensure you incorporate more oily fish such as salmon, trout or mackerel into your diet at least once a week, or whole eggs, milk, seeds and yoghurt.

Calcium – is required for maintaining strong bones, in addition to controlling nerve and muscle functions, making it essential for every cell in your body. Signs of deficiency include osteoporosis, fatigue, poor appetite, muscle cramps and abnormal heart rhythms. Although public perception often portrays milk as the best source, other options include dark leafy greens such as spinach, kale or broccoli, nuts and other dairy such as cheese or yoghurt.

Vitamin B12 – is used by every cell in your body, helps neurotransmitters in your brain, along with aiding in the production of DNA and red blood cells. Vitamin B12 is pretty much only found in animal products such as chicken, fish, shellfish, eggs and dairy, which means that vegetarians and vegans are highly susceptible to being deficient and if that applies to you, then it's highly recommended that you consider supplementation. Severe symptoms can include problems with walking or balance, numbness in the hands, legs or feet, anaemia, fatigue, paranoia, memory loss, or even hallucinations.

Potassium – is vital to help your heart, kidneys and other organs properly function, in addition to controlling fluid levels in the body. Illnesses which cause vomiting, diarrhoea or excess sweating can cause deficiencies and symptoms include weight loss, constipation and muscle weakness. The best sources include bananas, milk, vegetables, whole grains, peas and beans.

Iron – aids in producing red blood cells, meaning low levels make your body unable to effectively transport oxygen. Research shows that up to 25 percent of people are deficient in iron and symptoms include anaemia, fatigue and low levels of energy, along with possibly pale skin and sparse, thin dull hair. Much like Vitamin B12, vegetarians and vegans are particularly at risk and good sources include beef, beans, chickpeas, spinach and lentils.

Warning: Even with the high levels of people deficient in iron, it's something you should never supplement with. Too much can be very harmful and instead you should focus on getting enough through your diet.

Magnesium – supports bone health and the production of energy. While most healthy people are unlikely to be deficient, it can be a side effect of certain medications or associated with some health conditions due to issues with absorption. It can also be caused by over consumption of alcohol. Symptoms include nausea, vomiting, loss of appetite, anaemia, irregular heart rhythms and fatigue. Low levels of magnesium can also cause deficiencies of calcium and potassium in the blood. Good sources include spinach, black beans, whole grains, red meat and nuts.

Iodine – is essential for a normal functioning thyroid, due to its role in the production of various hormones and the most common symptom is an enlarged thyroid gland. Deficiencies are believed to affect up to one third of the world's population, and good sources include fish, yoghurt and eggs.

"The best and most efficient pharmacy is within your own system."
- Robert C. Peale

Supplements

There seems to be a supplement for everything these days, from boosting your immune system, to making your hair shinier, granting everlasting youth, or bringing about world peace. In fact, if there's a potential problem out there, then you can pretty much guarantee there's a pill-based solution for it, and even if it isn't a problem, there's no doubt someone trying to convince you it is, desperately trying to tell you what you want to hear, and trying even harder to sell you something you probably don't need.

In case you haven't already guessed, I'm not a big fan of supplements or the industry, and instead I'm a firm believer in trying to get everything we need from our diet, with as little man-made intervention as possible. Not only is this a more natural approach, but it's also far cheaper, with the added bonus of not having to fill your body with substances that are poorly regulated and often don't do anything more than make expensive urine. That's not to say there isn't a time and a place for supplements, or that they should all be branded with the same brush, as there definitely are some fantastic products out there that can and do make people's lives better, you just need to be careful who you trust and ensure that it is in fact something you actually need.

The supplement industry

The reality is the supplement business is a multi-billion dollar a year industry, with ginormous mark ups in prices and an astounding amount of manufacturers competing for a piece of the pie. In 2014 market research company Euromonitor International found that supplement sales are now worth more than $50 billion a year globally, and with the ever growing trends of health and fitness, this seems likely to continue increasing every year. It's just like any other business, where there are shareholders to please, interests to protect, and the ultimate goal of cutting costs and increasing profits. That's why you will often be paying more for marketing than anything else, with some estimations predicting that manufacturing costs can range anywhere from between a tenth to a twentieth of the retail price, with some unsurprisingly costing considerably more.

This holds especially true for big brands in named stores, as very few people are informed enough on the subject and therefore simply assume they are paying for what it's worth, with high street retailers making an absolute fortune from the unsuspecting consumer. To make matters worse, many products are simply a worthless waste of money. Yes, you read that right, a worthless waste of money. Many of the studies conducted or cited for products claiming to be 'scientifically proven' were funded by the very people producing them, with research often only conducted on rats or in other tests, and not actually on humans. Not only that, but they are often produced with cheap ingredients at ineffective dosages, then packaged in a way that promises miracle cures or results, with ridiculously expensive endorsements to try and buy trust. Then they are flogged to the unsuspecting consumer, who is simply trying to take positive measures to improve their health, oblivious to the fact that in all likelihood their good intentions are simply being exploited.

Multivitamins are often the worst culprits, as producers will often fill space with cheaper ingredients and only put in tiny amounts of more expensive ones, simply to say that they are included, and not coming anywhere near clinically effective dosages. The problem with this is that the cheaper ingredients are what we commonly have an abundance of in our diet already, whereas the more expensive ingredients are often what we are trying to avoid being deficient in and may even be what misled us into buying the product in the first place.

Muscle building and weight loss supplements are even worse, as the market is filled with products from fat burners to amino acids and testosterone boosters, all of which make huge outlandish claims of their life changing influences and how they will transform your body into a Greek God overnight, skipping all the hard work that's actually required and unsurprisingly, most effectively do nothing. Yet with no real regulations or governing body watching over them, these products are easy to sell due to the unsuspecting consumer buying into the hype, looking for any glimpse of hope that will make their goals easier to achieve.

The 'placebo' effect

You have no doubt heard of the placebo effect, but what you may not know is that it's been scientifically proven to exist. What this means is that by simply believing in the effectiveness of a product, supplement or medicine, can in some instances, actually make it work. There are cases of people curing all forms of illness imaginable, overcoming everything from depression to anxiety, lowering blood pressure, diabetes, heart disease and even cancer. You name it and there will no doubt be someone who swears by the therapeutic value of these products, when in fact, they have little to no effect at all. The reason why this happens is because the human body is capable of tremendous things, from healing to treating, or even reversing diseases. But a huge aspect that is often overlooked is how much of an influence our mindset has on its ability to effectively perform these tasks, and the fact that during desperate times people will believe in or cling to anything that offers a glimmer of hope. This state of mind can thereby convince them this 'miracle cure' will make everything better, which in turn, actually works, as it's pushed them to overcome the biggest barrier of them all – their mind.

Still not convinced?

As you have already seen, by having a more positive mindset you place less stress on your body, reducing the impact of hormones such as cortisol, which can often shut down various processes, such as your immune system. This in part explains why by simply believing that a product will work, can give the user the mental boost into believing it has, as this belief aids in directly helping them avoid going into 'fight or flight mode', along with all the negative connotations involved with entering this state too regularly.

That's not to say that all supplements are bad and there

definitely is a place for their use in a balanced lifestyle, especially for those who are unable to successfully get what they need from their diet, such as vegans, vegetarians or people with food intolerances. There are some fantastic companies out there who really do care about their products and the health of their consumers, but as with anything else, you really do need to be careful about who you trust and believe.

Making more informed decisions

When deciding whether or not to purchase a supplement, make sure you thoroughly read the back, looking at the RDA's (recommended daily amounts) and using that as the deciding factor in your purchasing decision. It's definitely worth doing some research on exactly what you are buying before parting with your hard earned cash, and there are a few trustworthy resources online that independently verify exactly what's in certain products, such as Examine.com or Consumer Lab.

While personally I try and avoid taking supplements, there are a couple of exceptions, as I do take Vitamin D and Omega 3. This is simply because of how difficult they can potentially be to get enough of in my diet, and I would rather be safe and avoid any potential deficiencies. This is a perfect example of working out what my body needs, and making an informed decision from there. With that being said though, I'm in no way prescribing or telling you what you should or shouldn't do, as it's entirely possible to avoid all deficiencies, without having to take supplements, under normal and healthy circumstances. On the other side of that, if they are something that work for you and you choose to consume, then there's nothing wrong with that either. Just always remember, if a product sounds too good to be true, then chances are it probably is and supplements should be used and treated as exactly what they are – supplements. Which means they should be used as a tool to support a balanced diet, rather than in place of it.

Fibre

Fibre is a carbohydrate found solely in plant foods such as vegetables, fruits and whole grains, where it's primarily concentrated in the skin, membrane and seeds. Even though it holds no magical fat burning properties, fibre is one of the unsung heroes when it comes to a healthy diet and weight loss.

What's so special about fibre?

Fibre is essential for maintaining a healthy digestive system and when consumed helps fill your stomach, thereby stimulating receptors that tell your brain when you have had enough. This helps stop over eating and aids in keeping you fuller for longer. Your body doesn't digest fibre easily either, which means that it's able to slowly pass through your system without spiking or causing blood sugar levels to rise. This is important as it allows you to maintain constant and steady energy levels throughout the day. Furthermore, by not spiking your blood sugar levels, less insulin is released into your bloodstream, which improves how your body responds to insulin, with the knock on effect of lowering your risks of both type 2 diabetes and heart disease. In addition, increased fibre intake has been linked to reducing the risk of other metabolic diseases, diverticulitis (intestinal inflammation) and some cancers.

Fibre comes in two forms:

Soluble fibre: which is what slows the breakdown of complex carbohydrates into glucose, causing reduced blood sugar levels in the blood. This gives the feeling of fullness and significantly reduces your appetite. Eating a diet high in soluble fibre has also been linked to a healthy heart, easier weight management, reduced cholesterol levels in the blood, as well as fat around the organs. Good sources include oats, potatoes, rye, barley, pulses, fruits and vegetables.

Insoluble fibre: doesn't dissolve in water and isn't digested or absorbed by your body. Therefore, it aids in keeping your gastrointestinal tract clean and allows for regular bowel movements by making it easier for stools to pass. Insoluble fibre is found naturally in wholemeal bread, brown rice, seeds, pulses, wholegrain cereals, and in the skins of fruits and vegetables.

The USDA recommends that adults have around 14 grams of fibre for every 1000 calories they consume, yet studies have found that the average diet in the Western World contains only half of that. This is largely down to the fact that when foods are processed or refined, the fibre is removed and its exclusion can be linked to both the obesity and chronic disease epidemics. From a nutritional standpoint, it is incredibly beneficial to increase our fibre intake, especially since this has the added benefit of directly increasing your intake of fruits and vegetables. Increasing fibre intake on a wholefoods diet is easy, as by simply eating healthier foods you will be increasing your intake without the need to track or worry about how much is in them. It is however important to remember that peeling fruits and vegetables drastically reduces their fibre content, meaning it's best to eat them whole wherever possible.

"Water is the most neglected nutrient in your diet, but one of the most vital."

- Julia Child

Water and avoiding dehydration

Your body comprises of around two thirds water, so you probably won't be surprised to hear that consuming enough is essential for both improving and sustaining your health. Along with eating more fruit and vegetables, drinking more seems to be one of the most regularly thrown around pieces of advice, yet research shows that only one in four people in the UK and one in three in the States are listening and drinking enough on a daily basis.

Water plays a role in influencing everything from your energy levels to helping your heart pump blood more effectively, regulating body temperature, aiding with digestion, keeping you regular, nourishing your skin, along with transporting nutrients and oxygen to your cells, making it pretty much essential for almost every function throughout your body. In fact, while you can survive for up to a month without food, you would only last a week without water.

The less water in your body, the thicker your blood becomes, which in turn means your heart has to work harder to pump oxygen to your brain, muscles, organs and other cells. Everyday you lose water through various processes, such as sweating, breathing, urination or excreting faeces, which is why you need to ensure you continuously supply your body with adequate amounts in order to top up what is lost and avoid dehydration, which is simply what happens when the body loses more water than it takes in. As this gets worse it can initially lead to feelings or thirst, being irritable or having a headache, but in time it can quickly worsen to exhaustion, fatigue, being clumsy, uncoordinated and having poor motor functions. With more extreme cases developing into nausea, dizziness, vomiting and eventually death. Research has even found that a loss as small as one percent can have a noticeable effect on exercise performance, with two percent impairing mental performance and around ten percent being potentially fatal.

How much do you need?

Most health authorities recommend that the average person has around two litres, or eight glasses a day. While these baseline recommendations for two litres a day are fine, they are very much general guidelines and this amount can fluctuate heavily depending on factors such as activity levels, surrounding environmental conditions, body composition and lifestyles choices. For instance, people involved in exercise or living in warmer climates require higher intakes, due to increased losses through sweating. As everyone is different, determining how much you need will very much be a case of listening to your body and seeing how it responds.

With that in mind, what are the signs of dehydration?

If you are feeling thirsty then it's a pretty good indication that you are already dehydrated, with another sign being the colour of your urine. A light yellow/straw colour indicates you are sufficiently hydrated, whereas the darker the shade, the bigger the sign that you need substantially more water in your system.

Where do you get water from?

Most people think water intake revolves purely around what they drink, but you get a substantial amount from your diet, with fruits and vegetables both being excellent sources. For instance, a medium banana contains 90ml of water!

Foods high in water can aid in preventing overeating, making drinking enough one of the most overlooked tools in both losing and maintaining weight. A perfect example of this is you will no doubt find you have no problem finishing a bag of cookies, whereas you may struggle with the last few pieces of broccoli on your plate. Now before you go thinking that's because cookies are delicious and broccoli is less enticing, the actual reason why is that broccoli is about 95 percent water, thereby filling up far more of your stomach than the crumbs of the cookies.

Any other problems?

Dehydration is an issue many people are facing on a daily basis and it has clearly been linked to weight gain and contributing to poor dietary choices. This is because it's easy to confuse the feelings of thirst with hunger, meaning that failing to get sufficient water intake can have a huge impact on everything from your cravings, to what or how much you eat.

What can be done about it?

If you have problems with snacking or are trying to lose weight, one strategy you can use to see if you are truly hungry or just thirsty is to firstly drink a glass of water and wait 15 minutes to see if the feelings have passed. This may save you a substantial amount of excess calories everyday, as it may remove the desire to turn to that afternoon snack, which could have just been your body signalling it needed fluids. What's more, it gives you some time to fully decide if it's what you truly want, and by removing acting on instinct or on in the moment decisions, drinking water can in turn reduce choices made by temptation.

In fact, water is a much-underused tool in weight loss and another strategy to incorporate is to drink a glass of water about 15 minutes before every meal. This is because your stomach measures fullness based on the volume of what you have consumed and not the calories, so by having water beforehand you can partially fill your stomach, as well as ensure that the hunger is genuine, and not a result of dehydration. It's important to note that all beverages you consume count towards your daily requirements, but for health reasons it's best to stick to plain water or teas wherever possible.

Other strategies for increasing intake

Personally, I have found the easiest way to get people to keep track of their water intake is to get them to fill a water bottle in the morning, keep it with them at all times, and ensure it's finished by the end of the day. Another tactic is to start your day by drinking one to two glasses first thing in the morning when you get up. Not only will this help you wake up, but it will also kick start your body's functions, as it will have become dehydrated during the night. If you are prone to fizzy drinks or hot beverages, start small by swapping out every other drink. If plain water isn't your thing, then make it more interesting by drinking herbal, flavoured or green teas, adding some lemon, lime, orange or cucumber slices, or even some ginger, mint or a variety of other herbs and flavourings. Whatever you do though, try to avoid cordials or anything with high amounts of sugar, artificial sweeteners or any other empty calories such as juice or soda.

Considerations for exercising

For every hour of exercise undertaken, you should be looking to add a further one to one and a half litres of water depending on the intensity at which you performed. With the Journal of Nutrition advising that for every 10 to 20 minutes of moderate exercise, an additional 200ml to 285ml should be consumed. That's why it's a good idea to always keep a water bottle with you when engaging in activity so that it's on hand throughout.

Gluten

It seems that going gluten free is all the rage these days and unless you've been living under a rock, you've no doubt in one way or another been inundated with products, gurus and pieces of advice, all naming and shaming glutens inclusion in our diet. Even though it's not a nutrient that's vital for health, I felt that because of the current gluten free dieting craze sweeping the nation, it needed to be included in this section to clear up any confusion or misunderstanding in regards to what you should be doing. Like most dieting trends, many people hop on the bandwagon with something they are told or led to believe. After all, if all the celebrities are doing it, then surely there must at least be some substance behind all these miraculous claims?!

People everywhere are stating that removing gluten from your diet helps a vast amount of conditions both mentally and physically. From easing bloating to clearing your skin, improving digestion or unlocking magical superpowers that are being locked up every time you reach for that slice of bread. There seems to be no problem that can't be solved by simply removing foods containing gluten from your diet and at this rate I wouldn't be surprised if next it's hailed as the saviour that's finally going to bring about world peace.

But is gluten really the enemy it's made out to be?

Let's cut straight to the point. No it's not, and I'm sorry if this comes across as condescending, belittling or even sarcastic, but as you can no doubt guess, I'm hugely against this entire craze, as it's simply gotten completely out of control. The reality is fad diets and products capitalise on finding something they can point the finger at and blame for health and weight problems, simply because it's easy to sell and the issue at hand is no exception. It's even reached the ridiculous extent where supermarkets are littered with products labelled as 'gluten free'. Most of which don't and never have contained gluten in the first place, such as fruits, vegetables, dairy, or a whole host of other items. But by simply whacking a sticker on them, they can take advantage of the health conscious consumer and this has become a simple way to shift a tremendous amount of everyday products, at an often elevated price.

I actually despair at the amount of people I have encountered who have said they are going gluten free, as when asked why, most can't give a single valid reason in regards to their decision, apart from because they have been told to do so. To make matters worse, most seem to have no clue what gluten actually is, so before you jump ship and make the same mistake, let's get serious for a minute and take a look at it in a little more detail.

What is Gluten?

Gluten is a protein that naturally occurs in wheat products, along with other grains such as barley, spelt and rye. While it's true that there are some health risks where it causes autoimmune responses for those with Celiac Disease, the reality is the amount of people it affects is relatively small in number. In fact, it's estimated that Celiac Disease affects between 0.3 to 1.2 percent of the population, yet studies in the UK have shown that more than one in five people have self-diagnosed themselves as having a gluten intolerance! Research conducted at Portsmouth University found that in reality, only two percent of them actually do, which in itself is pretty clear evidence that this entire craze has been massively and unnecessarily blown out of proportion.

What are the symptoms of gluten intolerance?

These can range from anything to do with gastrointestinal bloating to diarrhoea, flatulence, headaches, muscle pain and fatigue. However, these symptoms can be caused by a whole host of other food related intolerances, from dairy to certain types of carbohydrates, additives or even intestinal gas build up brought on by foods such as beans or cabbage. Meaning that what people are interpreting as a gluten insensitivity, is in all likelihood being caused by something else altogether.

Still not convinced?

Well in 2013 a study conducted by Monash University found in participants with self-reported non-celiac gluten sensitivity that negative symptoms were only caused when those involved knew they were eating gluten. They actually found that when they were led to believe they were consuming something else, that no symptoms were experienced. Showing a complete placebo effect in play. It was found that gastrointestinal issues weren't improved by reducing gluten intake from participant's diets, but what did have a positive effect was reducing the amount of fermentable, poorly absorbed, short-chain carbohydrates, which are more commonly referred to as FODMAPS. These are often found in grains, dairy, beans and some fruits, which coincides with other studies that suggest that what many people believe to be a sensitivity to gluten, is actually down to FODMAP's instead.

That means it's not gluten causing the problems, but rather these carbohydrates that aren't absorbed by the small intestine, instead passing into the large intestine and creating gas, bloating or discomfort when fermented by bacteria. With more severe circumstances leading to fatigue, headaches, lethargy and constipation. Thereby concluding that these symptoms are in fact caused by irritable bowel syndrome, and not down to gluten.

The problem however is that often many gluten based foods also contain these FODMAP's, which in turn has played a huge role in why it's taken the brunt of the miss focus. So if you are experiencing any of these side effects, chances are your body may just not respond well to certain foods and gluten itself has nothing to do with the issues. With that being said though, if you are having negative reactions or discomfort then obviously in these cases it makes sense to avoid foods causing the problems. So if a food makes you feel uncomfortable, try removing it from your diet for a week and see if the feelings subsist. If they do, then chances are that something within that product is the culprit and it's best to avoid or minimise its intake in the future.

For the majority of people there really is no need to adapt to a gluten free diet and doing so can actually bring about many other problems. For instance, while going gluten free is currently being portrayed as 'healthy', the alternatives people use as replacements are often far less nutritious carbohydrates, many of which contain less fibre, are higher in fat and lower in protein!

From a health perspective, completely removing gluten can actually have various drawbacks, as research has shown it's common for people with Celiac Disease to have various micronutrient deficiencies. This is because a gluten free diet can potentially prevent them from getting the full range of nutrients they require, a common factor associated with all restrictive diets. At the same time though, you shouldn't go overboard with gluten consumption and instead should limit it to a few times a week. It's just like anything else, where it's all about balance and consuming too much of anything can have negative connotations. Like with all dieting trends, things are never quite as black and white as they claim to be and chances are if it sounds too good to be true, then it probably is. This is why you should always face the issues with a certain degree of scepticism.

Chances are there really is no need for you to remove gluten from your diet and instead what you should be focusing on is listening to your body and seeing how it responds to the foods you consume, as that's the only true sign of what you really need.

Alcohol

While most of us like a drink from time to time, just like overindulging in food, we are all well aware of the health risks involved. Alcohol abuse has the potential to affect not only our body, but our lifestyle as well, with overconsumption and binge drinking becoming a huge problem in our society. The risks include everything from brain injury to memory loss, black outs and anxiety, with long-term abuse leading to serious mental health issues, permanent brain damage, in addition to alcohol dependence and alcoholism. Not only that, but it can also affect our sleep, blood pressure, appearance, and cause irreversible damage to our liver and other organs.

When you look at the bigger picture, alcohol use is not that dissimilar from what we discussed in the relationships with food section, as it is often turned to in times of distress, and used as a coping mechanism or measure of seeking comfort in circumstances we can't control. It regularly takes centre stage in countless movies and TV shows, turned to during difficult times as a form of relief, and portrayed as a magical liquid that can soothe everything from fear to doubt, anxiety, depression, conflict, or any other negative emotions. On the other side of that, it's use is often linked to celebration, playing a central part in everything from family holidays to sporting events and graduations, or even just as a way to relax and unwind at the end of long day.

There's no denying that alcohol use is a touchy subject, especially since it's not my place to be telling you what you should or shouldn't do. That's why instead I'm going to take the discussion back to the issue at hand, which is how it influences dieting and weight loss.

You will probably be pleased to hear that in small amounts there are potential health benefits from consuming alcohol, such as improved insulin sensitivity, how your heart functions, along with reduced blood lipids (fatty substances found in the blood that when lowered reduces the risk of heart disease). In fact, there's actually various studies which have found that moderate amounts of alcohol can potentially have a positive effect on losing weight. In 1958 the American Journal of Clinical Nutrition studied the diets of 1,944 adults who were aged between the ages of 18 to 74. They found that increasing calories from alcohol by itself didn't result in the same amount of weight gain as would be expected if those calories came from protein, carbohydrates or fats. Due to the regular consumption of alcohol, the drinkers were taking around 16 percent more calories everyday than non-drinkers, doing the same levels of activity, yet weren't any fatter than those who didn't consume alcohol. This topic was explored even further in another study, who put a group of obese woman on a weight loss diet, with one group getting 10 percent of their daily calories from white wine, while the other got it from grape juice. After three months the white wine group had lost around two pounds more than the grape juice group.

How or why this happens still isn't perfectly clear, but it can be speculated that this is partly down to alcohol consumption reducing our appetite, or it may even be related to the effects it has on insulin sensitivity.

While that may come across as me giving you the green light on drinking, as with everything else the issue really isn't that black and white, and alcohol consumption can in fact indirectly hinder your weight loss efforts. Even though alcohol can't be stored as body fat, the problems occur with how it blocks fat oxidation. What this means is that it slows down how quickly your body can break down dietary fat, and in turn accelerates the rate at which it is stored as body fat. Basically, the calories from alcohol aren't what causes us to gain weight, it's all the questionable food we choose to consume alongside it, which let's be honest, foods like kebabs, fried chicken and pizza become far harder to resist after a few drinks.

The bottom line is that the inclusion of alcohol is in no way necessary for our health, and while there's nothing wrong with having the occasional drink, if you are serious about improving your health and achieving your weight goals, then alcohol use does need to be kept within moderation.

If you are going to be drinking, then there are a few strategies you can use to minimise the damage to your waistline:
- Keep your dietary fat intake low for that day, and make sure you don't eat any fatty foods while you are drinking.
- Aim to get most of your calories for that day from protein and carbohydrates, with protein making up the bulk of what you consume.
- Try and avoid carbohydrate based beverages such as beer or fruity drinks. Dry wines or spirits are a far better alternative, again though be careful with what you mix them with.

These strategies will allow you to have a few drinks each week, without having to feel guilty or messing up your weight loss. As with everything you choose to do, it's all about balance, as there is place for everything in a healthy lifestyle.

"Some things you have to do every day. Eating seven apples on Saturday
night instead of one a day just isn't going to get the job done."

- Jim Rohn

What nutrition principles should you be following?

Dr. David Katz from Yale University's Prevention Research Center claimed: "A diet of minimally processed foods close to nature, predominantly plants, is decisively associated with health promotion and disease prevention."

Simply put; in order to achieve optimal health and reduce your risk of developing disease, you should be aiming to consume a diet based primarily around whole, unprocessed foods, that are as close to their original form as possible. To achieve this, you ideally want to be consuming meals consisting of different ingredients from these sources and avoiding processed foods containing heavily refined products wherever possible. You also need to be keeping your diet varied, as that way you can ensure you get the complete range of nutrients you require.

It's easy to interpret that as overly complicated and meaning the rest of your life will revolve around eating "rabbit food", or spending hours everyday cooking, but don't panic, as that's not even remotely true. Following a mostly wholefoods diet is far easier than you think and with a little thought and planning can be both convenient and delicious. If this way of eating is new to you, then I completely understand it can be a daunting or frightening concept, something you are hesitant to try or even convinced you won't enjoy. Initially it may just take some preparation and experimenting to determine what foods you enjoy, how to incorporate them into your meals and studying food labels to get an understanding of exactly what you are buying. But this is a minor inconvenience when compared to the huge health benefits gained and once you get the hang of it, it will become just another part of your daily routine. You just need to remember that just like any other new pursuit it takes some time, patience and a bit of work to get used to, so don't be put off if the processes are slow at first. I know this may potentially be a huge change that you need to adapt to and that's OK. At the end of the day, you are looking to make changes that will last a lifetime, meaning small steps are still progress, and as long as you are moving forward it doesn't matter how long it takes you to get to where you want to be. Trust me when I say that your initial fears and doubts as to whether or not you can do this, or concerns over what you perceive to be giving up will pass, especially as you start to see and feel the benefits of your actions.

"We are living in a world today where lemonade is made from artificial flavours and furniture polish is made from real lemons."
- Alfred E. Newman

Processed food

Before going any further, I firstly want to clear up any confusion as to what exactly I mean when I talk about reducing your intake of processed food. Processed food is a term thrown around and demonised in most fad diets, as it's far easier to pitch and sell someone on an idea when you have a clear target or enemy to point the finger at and blame for all their problems. Nevertheless, most of these diets completely disregard what actually constitutes processed foods, pigeonholing them as all being the same and the way in which I have discussed them so far in this book could no doubt be criticised for doing exactly the same thing. I have however purposely left clearing up any confusion over what I truly mean until now, as it's here that the issue can be treated as a centrepiece, rather than getting over shadowed by other ideas or being loosely defined and lost.

Processed food can be categorised as any product that has been altered in any way, shape or form from its original state. Meaning many processed foods are in fact staples in a healthy diet and have a vast amount of nutritional value. With just a few examples including Greek yoghurt, milk, nut butters, cheese, along with tinned or frozen fruits and vegetables. In fact, even fruits and vegetables placed in plastic bags could in a way be considered as processed, as they have gone through a procedure to get them to the point of sale. So with that being said, when I talk amount reducing your intake of processed foods, I'm saying you need to be choosing options that are minimally refined, without added sugar, hydrogenated oils and not filled with unwanted chemicals, preservatives, additives or artificial sweeteners.

However, with how hectic life has become there will always be times when convenience will become the deciding factor in your decisions, and it's completely unrealistic to say that you should never eat something that comes out of a box or container again, which is why I'm not even going to ask you to try. Instead it's important that you start paying attention to what products are made of, as this will enable you to make more informed decisions on what you put into your body, and reduce the amount of toxins you consume. This is especially true when there are several options of similar products available, as while you may not be able to completely remove them from your diet, you can at least determine which of them is likely to do the least harm. It may not seem like much, but if you are regularly making the best choice available, then in the long run all those small reductions in toxins will add up and have a hugely positive impact on your health.

Be that as it may, I don't think there's anything wrong with still consuming heavily processed foods, as long as you only do so occasionally, say once or maybe sometimes twice a month. As I said before, I still like indulging in the occasional burger, pizza or slice of cake, so it would be completely hypocritical to preach that you need to completely stop. Nonetheless, if your primary source of food intake comes from heavily processed sources, then that's where there's definitely cause for concern. That's why you need to transition into a healthier way of eating, taking small baby steps if needed and aiming to change both your habits and your mindset in regards to how you view and use food.

What is a calorie?

A calorie is a unit of energy and in everyday terms these are most commonly referring to the energy we consume through eating and drinking. From a more scientific perspective though, one calorie is the amount of energy required to increase one gram of water by one degree Celsius.

You have probably been told in the past that dieting and weight loss comes down to calories in versus calories out, essentially meaning that if you burn more than you take in, then you will lose weight and vice versa. In principle yes this is true, however from a health perspective, the reality really isn't that simple. Let's find out why.

Is a calorie a calorie?

A professor at Kansas University conducted a study to see if calorie counting was the primary factor that influenced success in terms of weight loss, and his findings shed

some interesting light towards answering this question. For ten weeks he lived on a convenience store diet, comprising of mostly Twinkies, Doritos, sugary cereals and other high sugar refined snacks. As many of these items contain little to no protein, he did however add in some protein shakes to ensure his intake didn't drop too drastically below unsafe levels. Before the study his daily intake was around 2,600 calories, so during the ten weeks he limited it to 1,600 calories. By the end of the period he had lost

27 pounds, and reduced his body fat percentage from 33.4 to 24.9 percent.

But wait what?! Doesn't that go against everything I have told you so far?

You may suddenly be thinking if that's all it takes, then why bother with all the healthy eating and lifestyle changes? Surely that study is counterproductive to the message I'm trying to get across? Proving a calorie is a calorie, regardless of the source you get it from? Well as I have stressed throughout this book, this isn't simply about losing weight. It's about developing a healthy and sustainable lifestyle, where you not only look good, but also feel good as well, with weight loss being a positive side effect of the process and the changes that you make.

The point I am trying to make is that while he may have lost weight in the study, his success was very much at the expense of his wellbeing and if he continued in this manner then it would only be a matter of time before it took a toll on his health. While this may seem like an 'extreme' example, the sad reality is that his experiment is actually similar to the standard way that many people eat on a daily basis. The major difference though is they aren't doing it within a controlled environment, and there's no set end date or calorie restriction either. In fact, the only reason why he lost weight was due to eating 1600 calories a day, which is below what was required to maintain his weight.

Research has shown that people who have diets based primarily around processed foods are regularly consuming substantially more calories than they require. That's because if you look at it properly, 1600 calories is quickly filled by a couple of chocolate bars and bags of cookies, a mere fraction of the amount of food you would need to feel full on a daily basis. Meaning through the duration of this study he really was starving himself, both physically and nutritionally, making it not even remotely maintainable long-term.

Why is a calorie not a calorie?

While in essence all calories are the same in regards to having the same amount of energy, the reality of the matter is the human body is a complex biochemical system. This means that what you eat has a huge impact on the processes involved in metabolising the nutrients, as the responses and hormones triggered vary depending on the food consumed. Simply put, the way your body reacts to foods is substantially different depending on what you eat. Not only that, but there exists something called the 'thermic effect' of food, which is a measurement of how much energy is expended in breaking food down, as the amount needed to digest, absorb and metabolise the nutrients varies considerably. For instance, protein requires far more energy to process than carbohydrates or fats.

The food you eat can directly affect everything from how you store fat to your cravings, gut flora, how your liver responds, as well as your glucose, insulin and hormone responses. While technically in terms of the chemistry behind it all a calorie is a calorie, in the grand scheme of things, they are far from equal. On top of that, 100 calories from whole food sources such as vegetables affects your body in a very different way than 100 calories from processed sources such as chocolate or soda. Even more, just by looking at how much 300 calories of healthy food looks like to 300 calories of chocolate, pastry or chips, you will clearly see a winner in the portion size that is likely to fill you up.

"By failing to prepare, you are preparing to fail."
- Benjamin Franklin

Reading food labels

There is definitely a huge misconception about people who spend time reading food labels, portraying them as pedantic and overly obsessed with every calorie they consume. But have you ever actually looked at the ingredients in the everyday items you consume? Many people believe they are following a healthy diet, oblivious to the fact that many of the products they are purchasing are filled with so many additives, sugars, preservatives and other ingredients, that they are unknowingly poisoning their bodies. It may seem like hassle or like going over the top at first, but looking at food labels is the only way to get a better understanding of what you are actually eating. If you think about it properly, once you do it for the products you regularly purchase, you don't have to do it again, making it a one-off inconvenience, that has huge long-term health ramifications.

Doing so involves more than just looking at the numbers, as the calorie and macronutrient counts don't even come close to telling the whole picture, especially when legally these figures can be up to 25 percent off from the stated amounts. You also shouldn't take any notice of the health claims on the front of the box, as it's common practice for manufacturers to use misleading terms or false marketing promises and they will often do or say anything to convince you to buy their product over a competitor's. A perfect example of this is when Kellogg's released a 'protein' version of their popular Cheerio's cereal, a product which actually contained less than one gram more protein per equivalent serving size of the original, yet it had 17 times more sugar!

What to look for instead

Start by shifting your focus to the ingredients list on the back. These are listed in order of weight/amount, making the first two or three the most important to consider, as they are featured in the highest quantity and what the product is primarily made of. A good rule to follow when you are short on time, or don't want to study every label is to scan for what the first three ingredients are, as at least that way you have a good idea about what you are consuming. Alternatively, if you know what you are buying beforehand you could even check it out online on the store or manufacturers website at a time that's convenient. That way your shopping trip doesn't turn into an endless mission of reading boxes when you are in a rush and this is often what I tend to do when planning meals with new ingredients.

Ideally you want to be avoiding products where the first ingredients are refined grains, sugar or processed oils, as well as featuring ingredients you either don't know, or that don't sound like actual foods. Simply put, if the back of the box reads more like a science textbook, with a never-ending list of chemicals that you can't pronounce, then don't buy the product unless you desperately want it, or have no other alternative. It's no doubt been made in a lab to keep it fresh and extend its shelf life, with the added extras more likely than not offering a whole host of potential risks, without adding any nutritional value or health benefits. I'm not even exaggerating this issue either, as it has been found to be common practice for manufacturers to include chemicals in products that if you knew what they were, you wouldn't want anywhere near your body. For instance, Subway were found to be using a bleaching agent in their bread called azodicarbonamide, which is a chemical that's found in yoga mats. After a huge amount of controversy over the chemicals use, in 2014 they announced that they were in the process of removing the chemical from their products. While that is a step in the right direction, it's important to note that it's also widely used in products at other chains such as McDonalds, Starbucks and even breads sold at supermarkets.

Serving sizes

It's essential to look at the difference between a serving size and the total volume within the package, as it's easy to misinterpret or misjudge. A recommended serving size is often far less than you would expect or tend to use for one portion, making it easy to consume more than the amount intended. This is especially true for products such as cheese, peanut butter, or anything else out of a tub or jar. The back of the package usually lists the nutritional information per 100 grams, along with the recommended serving size, or depending on the product, its entire contents. Always keep that in mind, as it's common practice for manufacturers to try and deceive consumers into believing their product is healthier than it is, by taking advantage of the fact that it's not common knowledge that a serving size doesn't actually mean the entire product. Meaning it could actually just be half that can of soda, a quarter of a chocolate bar, or a small corner of that block of cheese.

Other considerations

One of the main problems with misperceptions to healthy eating is it has led to a high demand for low fat and fat free products. The issue with this is fat is often what gives food its flavour and when removed can leave it tasting bland and horrible. In many cases this has caused manufacturers to seek out alternatives to improve the taste of their products, with sugar or artificial sweeteners often taking centre stage as the replacement. That's why you need to be careful when choosing these products, as often those low fat yoghurts, cheeses and other items marketed as good for you, are actually far unhealthier than the full fat variants.

Equally, be careful of anything claiming to be organic, natural, fruit flavoured, or containing no added sugar, as even if that's the case, it doesn't magically make the product healthy. It's common for these labels to be attached simply to make the product more appealing to the health conscious consumer, as what they are claiming it to be free of is regularly replaced by something just as bad, if not worse.

Traffic light system

Another aspect of food labels introduced to help consumers make more informed decisions is the red, amber and green traffic light system. While in principle they are a good idea and can help with making quick on the spot decisions, they can also be highly misleading and deter buyers from purchasing products that are actually extremely good for their health. For example, I have dealt with many clients who have feared eating fats, due to misperceptions that they will cause them to gain weight. Now when placed in a supermarket setting and seeing red labels on bags of nuts or olive oils, all this does is reinforce their misperceptions that this isn't a product they should be purchasing. So yes, while these products are high in fat, they are filled with healthy fats that should be incorporated more into their diet. Yet they wouldn't think twice about grabbing a carton of orange juice, which in reality is far more damaging to their health and waistline.

These are just some of the reasons why you should be looking to buy whole foods wherever possible, as by opting for products that are the ingredients, rather than consisting of ingredients, you don't need to study any labels or lists. That's because there are no added extras, as they are still in their natural form. Like I said before, it's perfectly understandable that it's not always possible to choose products in this way. When you do decide to go for a package product, just make sure you spend some time to determine which is the healthiest of the options available, as with most things there are likely to be a few possibilities from which you could choose.

Sugar

When reading food labels, probably the most important thing you need to look for is often the hardest to spot, and that's added sugar. Sugar goes by countless different names, many of which your average consumer is unlikely to recognise.

Some of the most common forms of sugar to look out for are; high fructose corn syrup, cane sugar, corn sweetener, honey, agave nectar, dextran, maltodextrin, malt syrup, maltose or evaporated cane juice.

Basically watch out for anything that ends in 'ose', or sounds remotely along the same lines. More often than not it's likely to be sugar in one form or another and even if it's not, it will still probably be a chemical you want to be avoiding anyway.

"I think it's one of the most important battles for consumers to fight: the right to know what's in their food, and how it was grown."

- Joel Salatin

Sugar

I think I have made the dangers posed by a diet high in added sugars pretty clear so far, but one of the main problems is most people don't actually realise how much they are consuming on a daily basis. It's not that sugar is inherently bad; in fact, in small doses, or when found in natural sources such as fruit it helps to provide your brain and muscles with a form of energy. However, just like everything else, it's over consumption of the processed variety that tends to be made of empty calories and no added nutritional value that you need to be careful of, yet that's the form which is primarily being consumed. Sugar seems to be continually finding ways to sneak into our diets, often in sources you wouldn't even suspect and in far higher amounts than you would imagine. If you look at food labels you will be shocked to find that there's added sugar in everything from bread to milk and fruit juices, flavoured yoghurts, cereals, granola bars, tinned fruit, pasta sauces, ketchup, salad dressings and even dried fruit! Leaving people completely unaware that the choices they have been led to believe are healthy, may in reality contain just as much added sugar as the 'unhealthy' alternatives.

A prime example of this is clever marketing campaigns have managed to convince consumers that smoothies are a great way to increase their daily intake of fruits and vegetables, portraying them as an easy way to get one of your five a day. While this may be true if you are making them yourself, the ones on offer in shops are a completely different story, with many containing just as much sugar as soda, and in some cases even more! For example, a 250ml serving of Coke contains 26.5g of sugar, whereas a Naked mango smoothie contains 30g in the same amount!

Our society seems to have become dependent on sugar and this is largely due to the influence it has on people's brains. Much like taking a drug, sugar causes the body to release the feel-good hormone dopamine and it has been found that it takes just 30 minutes to go from that sought-after sugar rush, to a full on sugar crash. This action simply spurs on addiction, as one of the side effects of regularly consuming products high in sugar is that your taste buds become trained to crave them even more, making it a vicious cycle of mixed feelings and emotions, that you are never able to sustain. It has been claimed that if sugar came into use 50 years ago like it has today, it would have been classified as a class 'A' drug, with scientific research even suggesting that sugar is eight times more addictive than cocaine!

What makes matters worse is that food manufacturers have capitalised on people's addiction, by increasing the amounts added to their products. By getting buyers hooked and consuming larger quantities, they are able to keep them coming back for more. This in turn allows for continual growth in sales, along with skyrocketing profits at the expense of plummeting health. More worrying still is the extent in which this has spread, with one study in the USA finding that more than 600,000 food products in super markets (which is around 80 percent) have added sugar!

The health risks associated with sugar are undeniable and without hesitation I would label it as the worst ingredient in the modern diet. Essentially what overconsumption is doing is robbing our bodies of proper nutrition, as excessive intake has been linked to everything from diabetes to hypertension, increased blood cholesterol, difficulties controlling blood sugar levels, increased fat storage, Alzheimer's, obesity and some forms of cancer. Many of these issues are even interrelated, with heart disease and stroke accounting for 65 percent of deaths among type 2 diabetics. And that's only the physical side of it! Sugar has been directly correlated to depression, higher rates of anxiety, insomnia, low energy levels, tiredness, hunger and difficulties coping with stress. It also increases inflammation, which directly affects the immune system's ability to function, making it more difficult to ward off illnesses and infection. That's not even including the weight gain and negative relationships with food people tend to develop either. Sugar has been linked to overeating due to how it scrambles the signals sent to our brains, where high levels of insulin making us unable to tell when or if we are full. In turn this causes the consumption of far more calories than actually required, and it can negatively influence the food choices we make as well. A study out of Los Angeles University in California found that sugar creates what they termed as 'brain fog', suggesting that it compromises mental functions, such as your memory and learning. This makes it harder to focus on the present, affects your cognitive abilities and attention span, in addition to causing difficulties remembering the past.

Sugar and cancer

If the risks associated with excessive sugar intake weren't bad enough, research has shown that sugar feeds cancer cells, as glucose acts as a fuel allowing them to thrive and spread. This is because cancer cells tend to have plenty of insulin receptors, therefore giving them a greater response rate than normal cells to insulin's ability to promote growth. While it's not necessary to completely remove sugar from your diet, in order to prevent, treat or in some cases even cure some forms of cancer, you should be aiming to drastically reduce your intake, aiming to keep it more in line with the daily recommended amounts, and ideally keeping it even lower if possible. This will allow your body to more effectively control blood glucose levels, with the benefit being that it strengthens immune functions and starves cancer cells.

Whatever you do though, don't let this scare you into removing carbohydrates from your diet. This is a short sighted strategy people have turned to in a panic, in an attempt to control their glucose levels and is actually counterproductive to their health in a variety of ways. This is why you should instead be focusing on a wholefoods diet comprising of low GI sources wherever possible, so that sugar has a much more gradual infusion into the bloodstream, consequently placing far less stress on your body and reducing the negative impact that it has.

How much sugar should you be eating?

It's crazy to think that the average person has gone from eating ten pounds of sugar a year in 1800, to a staggering 152 pounds a year today! Because of that, the World Health Organisation has reduced their recommended daily intake amounts, stating that we should be getting no more than five to ten percent of our total calories from sugar, and ideally aiming for the lower end of that scale. Yet at present intake levels in the UK are estimated to be around 16 to 17 percent, and in America there are periods in time where consumption is thought to be close to double that amount.

How much should you be aiming for?

According to the guidelines, per day it works out to around 25g for women, which is approximately five to six teaspoons and 35g for men, which is about eight to nine teaspoons.

Keeping track of added sugar intake can get confusing, but the easiest way to work out how much is in a product is to look at the nutritional information table on the back of the box and divide the grams of sugar by four. That will give you the total number of teaspoons within the product and from there you can make a judgement call on your purchase. Again, make sure you are looking at the full amount you are likely to be consuming and not being misled by serving sizes.

Reducing your intake

From a health perspective there's no way around it, if you are truly serious about improving your wellbeing then reducing sugar intake is up there with ensuring you eat enough fruit and vegetables. I know it's difficult, especially since sugar is present in many of the foods we tend to eat on a daily basis, which is why I do understand that reducing your intake may be easier said than done, especially during the initial stages of adapting to a healthier way of eating. That's why instead of trying to cut it all out at once, you may be better off focusing on slowly reducing your intake wherever you can. This is because while your intentions may be in the right place, going cold turkey will inevitably just increase the stress you mentally and physically place on your body, causing withdraw symptoms, cravings and anxiety related to restriction. That's why instead it's best to try and make slow gradual changes, which depending on your current habits, could include anything from; swapping refined products such as white bread for wholegrain varieties, cutting down on the amount of sugar you add to drinks, replacing fruit juice with tea or water, making your own pasta sauces, choosing boxed items with the least sugar, or opting for plain yoghurt and adding your own fruit.

"Respect your body, and look forward to feeling healthy and clean. Your body deserves better than laboratory-made sweetness."

- Damon Gameau

Artificial sweeteners

I know I have spent the last few pages going on about sugar in a way that could be perceived as demonising it. No doubt leaving you searching for a bright light at the end of the tunnel to satisfy your sweet tooth, without all the added risks involved. But I'm sorry to be the barer of bad news, artificial sweeteners don't seem to be that magical solution, even though manufacturers have done an excellent job of portraying and marketing them as a miracle replacement. They have quickly become a staple part of many people's diets and can now be found in a wide variety of 'sugar free' products, with their rise in popularity in many ways down to promises of helping people lose weight. While I get the appeal of having a low, if not calorie free alternative to sugar, the reality is that even though some of these products have been approved as safe for human consumption, the health risks associated with their use are still widely disputed and unknown.

It seems that the experts can't even come close to agreeing on this issue either, as the overall effect they have still isn't fully understood. To make things even more confusing, the results shown in studies have varied widely, with some resulting in weight loss, some having a neutral effect, and others even showing weight gain. What findings do however suggest is that their use can be linked to increased appetite levels, which leads to an increase in food consumption and explains the cases where weight gain occurred, with these effects being known since as far back as the 1980's. An argument can however be made that the evidence presented in these cases was merely correlational, and that those using the highest amounts of sweeteners may actually have a predisposition for weight gain and overeating. For that reason, the likelihood is the effect they had may potentially have been highly dependent on the individual who consumed them, and how their body responded.

The truth of the matter is that at this present point in time we simply don't know enough about sweeteners to make an informed enough decision on their use and because of that it's one of those situations that for me anyway, doesn't seem worth the risk until further scientific evidence and research has been conducted. Especially since there are several claims linking their use to various cancers and other illnesses, with the evidence used in support of their consumption being questionable at best.

However, what is known and the reason why I personally try to avoid them as much as possible is that when you think about food your brain responds accordingly by getting your body ready for the nutrients it's about to receive. It does this so that it can efficiently put them to use and this is done by preparing your body to regulate your metabolism, weight, energy and burn calories, along with all the other various processes involved. So when your body tastes something sweet, it triggers the relevant metabolic and hormonal responses to deal with what is being consumed. This is where the problems occur, as even though they don't contain sugar, they still cause the body to respond in the same way by affecting your response to insulin, in turn raising insulin levels in your blood and because of that it can be speculated that they can come with the same metabolic risks.

On top of that, a new theory of how we process sugar has emerged, arguing that sweeteners (of any nature) could potentially deactivate the way our brain understands food. This is because naturally when receiving sugar your brain understands a calorific load coming along with it. On long-term sweetener consumption, the argument is that our brains might simply press the restart button on the sweet taste, "forgetting" that sweet = calories, meaning that it does not understand that when sugar is received, calories are received as well. The issue with this is that all the other processes affected by sugar are deactivated, making the body more likely to store fat, along with all the other metabolic risks that come with it. This concept is still very much in the theoretical stage, with an insufficient amount of evidence to say for certain as to whether or not this is in fact what happens. Be that as it may, it's still worth thinking about, especially when considering the long-term implications of our actions.

Just like sugar it's common for artificial sweeteners such as aspartame, sucralose or saccharin to be hidden under various different names within everyday products, which is why you need to be careful of anything claiming to be 'sugar free'. Chances are these substances will be used as a replacement of sugar, which is why you need to properly read food labels to get a better idea of what you are consuming.

Due to the lack of conclusive evidence there's no need to stress over or completely avoid their use, but in all likelihood you are far better off not turning to artificial sweeteners as a guilt free alternative and limiting their use wherever possible. With all that being said though, not all artificial sweeteners are created equal, and there is some new research suggesting that Stevia may actually be a healthy alternative. This is down to the fact it's 100 percent natural and is made directly from plants. At this present point in time, Stevia is still pretty new to the market and because of that, it's use in everyday products is fairly limited. Meaning that an abundance of products are still being produced with the forms you should be looking to avoid, with aspartame coming top of the list of products I won't go anywhere near. The jury on Stevia is still very much out though and there isn't enough evidence to make a solid judgement on the potential health risks it may hold.

Final thoughts

If you desperately want something sweet, stick to having a bit of sugar or honey instead. I know after everything I have said so far that may sound like the polar opposite to the advice you were expecting, but at least that way your body can respond accordingly, rather than receiving and trying to deal with mixed signals. Either way, you should be looking to reduce both your intake of both artificial sweeteners and sugar wherever you can.

How to put together a balanced diet

"When diet is wrong medicine is of no use. When diet is correct medicine is of no need."
- Ancient Ayurvedic Proverb

The purpose of this section is to clear up any confusion on how to put together a balanced diet, along with giving you all the knowledge and understanding of exactly how to apply it to your everyday life, without having to obsess over what you eat. It's my hope that by following the information laid out over the following pages, that you will be able to start making the transition towards a mindset of eating what your body truly needs, all while finally enjoying your food for what it is, without letting it take control of who you are.

I said right from the very start that traditional dieting methods based around restriction simply don't work, which is why you will find this approach to be very different from anything you have tried before. Whether you are looking to lose fat, build muscle or maintain your current weight, you will be able to take the principles discussed here and apply them directly to your circumstances.

You have probably already guessed that the majority of these principles revolve around eating natural, healthy foods, but that doesn't mean you will be sentenced to a life of dried out chicken and broccoli. One of the biggest misperceptions about eating healthier is that it can't be an enjoyable experience, and that's a mindset we need to work on changing right from the very start. Personally I love food, it's a huge part of my life and I refuse to accept the connotation that you have to sacrifice pleasure for health and can't have both.

You can use the ingredients discussed later to make healthy and delicious versions of any dish you can think of. From pasta to curries, burritos, burgers, pizzas or stir-frys, and these ingredients cover a whole range of dietary needs and cuisines. By finding a way to include everything you love, you won't have those feelings of missing out or giving something up, which is exactly why this way of eating is sustainable long-term.

To help people out with this change I have made it one of my goals to continuously put together healthy nutritious meals, that are quick and easy to make, all while most importantly, also delicious. These can be made by anyone, so whether you are new to cooking or a seasoned chef, you will be able to find recipes and inspiration based around a whole host of different foods on my website:

www.tailoredlifestyles.co.uk

Or on Facebook:

www.facebook.com/tailoredlifestyles

"In all aspects of our lives balance is key. Doing one thing too much can cause upset, like the old saying goes, everything in moderation is the secret!"
- Catherine Pulsifer

What is a balanced diet?

If just the thought of trying to eat healthier leaves you feeling lost and confused then don't worry, as you definitely aren't alone. At every turn we are told to eat a balanced diet, but the reality is, very few people seem to actually know what that means.

For me, a balanced diet is one that revolves around a variety of ingredients from primarily wholefood sources. These ingredients should be used to create meals you love, all while supplying your body with the full range of macro and micronutrients it requires to thrive, while still making room for the foods you love, but which are often deemed less beneficial to your health.

That's what balance is truly all about.

You have no doubt heard the term 'wholefoods' thrown around, but just like everything else it seems to have become an overused slogan adopted by advertisers to market products, leading to confusion and diversion over what it actually means.

So before we go any further, let's clear up that misinterpretation.

Wholefoods are nutrient-dense foods in their unrefined, original form and include vegetables, fruits, whole grains, legumes and soy products. These are all low in disease-causing substances and high in disease-preventing nutrients, which is why they should be forming the foundation on which a healthy diet is based. When these products are processed or refined, many of the nutrients they initially offered are either lost all together, or replaced with ingredients such as sugars, unhealthy fats, preservatives or other chemicals. For instance, when brown rice is refined into white rice it loses all of the fibre and bran, which are the components that keep you full, aid in digestion, help keep your blood sugar levels stable and curb hunger.

One of the main advantages of adopting a diet based primarily around wholefoods is the low calorie count in comparison to the total volume consumed. This is important as you can only eat so much until your stomach sends signals to your brain telling it you are full. Eating wholefoods makes it harder to overeat and reduces the chances of getting cravings or the desire to snack in-between meals. By eating mostly wholefoods, you will find that you are able to consume a far higher volume of food, while actually ingesting far fewer calories. Not only that, but studies repeatedly conclude that people who eat a diet of mostly low glycemic foods find it far easier to both lose and maintain their weight.

The reality is life is short, and while you should be doing everything you can to improve your health and longevity, you also need to enjoy yourself and make the most of the time you have. This is why in my opinion there are no 'good' or 'bad' foods. While it's undeniable that some foods are better for you than others, the reality is food is just food and the sooner you can get over this idea of labelling and shaming different products, the sooner you can remove the stigmas attached to eating, start making better decisions and improve your relationships with the foods you consume. We have talked quite a lot so far about how people's relationships with food are placing a huge strain on them mentally and emotionally, and it's this perception of products being good or bad that's directly contributing to this issue. Psychologically, as soon as you view a product as something you shouldn't be consuming, you start to feel guilty and develop detrimental attitudes and behaviours towards it. That's why it's absolutely essential that we get you to change your mindset in regards to how you both view and treat foods, as that will be the only way to positively start to progress in a sustainable manner.

Because of this, I recommend aiming to structure your intake to consist of around 80 to 90 percent nutritious foods, which still leaves room for products deemed less beneficial to your health. I know that sounds like a lot, but in the grand scheme of things it is a huge difference when compared to other 'diets' where they are completely off limits or removed. However, that doesn't mean you need to go off rushing around trying to find out what your daily calorie intake should be and frivolously working out what 10 to 20 percent of that would be in cookies. Instead, what it means is being more mindful of your consumption, and for the week as a whole aiming to reduce your treats to say one or two items, depending on their size or calorie content. There's no way around it, you simply can't keep consuming these items everyday and expect to achieve the health or weight you desire. Personally I try to save it for certain occasions, such as having dessert when out for a meal, or some chocolate or popcorn at the cinema. For you though this may mean still having a Friday night takeaway, or the occasional slice of cake. By eating in this manner nothing is ever off limits, but just remember it's all about balance and not going from one extreme to the other.

By eating this way there will be no more dieting, no more restriction, no more counting calories and definitely no more starving yourself. I don't know about you, but with all things considered, to me this approach seems like a more than reasonable compromise to make. I promise you that once you start to improve your eating behaviours in a way that doesn't revolve around restriction, you will have an easier time making more positive decisions, and the cravings for other items will start to disappear.

That's the difference between eating as part of a diet, or as a part of your life, as finding balance is the only way to make this maintainable long-term. Ultimately a diet's success shouldn't be measured by how you look after a few days or weeks, but instead should be based on how you look and feel after months or years. Always remember, this is all about lifelong health, which makes achieving that - the true testament as to how successful it actually is.

"Some people think the 'plant based whole foods diet' is extreme. Half a million a year will have their chests opened up and a vein taken from their leg and sewn onto their coronary artery. Some people would call that extreme'."

- Dr. B Caldwell

A different kind of 'diet'

Whenever I hear someone say the word diet, I immediately think of a set of rules or restrictions, based around doing something you don't want to do, but feel like you have to for a short period of time in order to try and lose weight. That's why I'm almost hesitant to use the word 'diet' when talking about this way of eating. But for lack of a better word, whenever 'diet' is used from this point forward, just remember I'm referring to the way you are aiming to start eating as part of your new healthier lifestyle.

For generations there have been changing government recommendations for what we should be consuming, and all this has done is spur on public misperceptions. The problem is that all the guidelines and models produced have been based on questionable evidence at best. I know that's a bold claim to make, but just think about the fact that if they were truly correct, year on year we wouldn't be facing a growing obesity and chronic disease epidemic. The issue at hand revolves around the fact that far too much focus is placed on isolating items into groups, rather than looking at the values and benefits different foods provide. That's why I have never understood how ideas such as the UK's Eat Well Plate have become so widely used and accepted, when their entire basis is inherently flawed. Instead, as an alternative to dividing everything into sections, there needs to be a concept or model that looks individually at the products within them, as that's the only way to determine accurately what you should or shouldn't be eating.

For instance, rather than saying 50 percent of calories should come from carbohydrates (which is meaningless advice without considering the sources they come from), the guidelines would be better if they recommended that 50 percent of calories came from complex, starchy or whole-grain carbohydrates, over refined variants. That's because there's a huge nutritional difference between getting 50 percent of your calories from wholefood sources such as oats, whole-wheat pasta and brown rice, as opposed to white bread, bagels and cereal. Yet, in most healthy eating models these products would fall into the same categories and this lack of distinction is what's leading many people astray. For example, while the Eat Well Model does recommend that you should be aiming to primarily consume starchy carbohydrates, the illustration used features them combined in the same section as refined variants. This in turn confuses consumers, as it promotes the idea that all carbohydrates are the same and therefore there is no difference between whether your intake is based on starchy or refined options. Let's be honest, most people simply go on what the picture shows and very few will take the time to properly read all the rules, suggestions and guidelines that come with them. I have even encountered someone who told me they had a balanced dinner because their pizza covered all aspects of the Eat Well Plate by having cheese for fat and dairy, beef for protein, peppers for vegetables and the base of the pizza being carbohydrates. While their judgment may seem absurd, if you look at it more closely and compare it to the pictures and dietary guidelines, logically, they aren't actually far off. That's why uttermost clarity on the differences of what we should actually be doing is absolutely essential, as that's the only way that people will start to become more aware and make better decisions.

This issue isn't helped by the fact that the experts can't even agree on what we should be eating either, but the good news is some progress was finally made in 2015, when the Dietary Guidelines Advisory Committee produced a report that at long last, is heading in the right direction. While there were a vast array of thoughts and opinions, this group of nutritional scientists did eventually come to a consensus about the core principles to follow in regards to putting together a balanced diet.

For optimum health, they suggested diets should be high in vegetables and fruit, whole grains, low or fat-free dairy, legumes, nuts and seafood. In addition, alcohol consumption should be kept to moderate levels and an effort made to lower intake of red and processed meats, refined grains, along with sugary foods and beverages. One thing I would like to throw into the mix is lean meats. Researchers on both sides of the argument massively debate the health risks and benefits of eating meat and I feel that because of the lack of concrete evidence either way, the decision should be left to you based on what you enjoy, as well as your preferences and beliefs. In the grand scheme of things, I'm not here to tell you what you can or can't do, I'm here to try and coach and guide you on making the best decisions for yourself as to what will most likely improve your health. Nevertheless, we should all be aiming to cut down on excessive portion sizes of meat, not just because of potential health reasons, but at the same time because of environmental issues such as our carbon footprint and the catastrophic damage that is being caused globally by mass farming animals.

"Don't eat anything your great-grandmother wouldn't recognize as food."
- Michael Pollan

What ingredients should you be using?

For a balanced diet it's essential you get a range of protein, carbohydrates and healthy fats to ensure you provide your body with the full range nutrients it requires to function properly. The best way to do this is to select a source of protein, carbohydrates and fat, along with a couple of servings of vegetables and flavourings for every meal. From these you will be able to make a version of any meal you desire. You should be aiming to eat one or two servings of fruit each day, which you can add in wherever best suits you. Obviously for most people vegetables won't be included in breakfast, but by adding two portions to lunch and dinner along with fruit, you will easily meet the five a day recommended amounts.

Over the following pages we will be looking at each of nutrients, along with the best sources to build your meals around. After that I'll give you some examples of how to apply this concept, and from there we can look at the bigger issue of putting it all together.

Protein

There's a vast amount of research linking a high protein diet to better health and for good reason. Protein is required by your body for various functions from growth to repair and producing hormones. Not only that, but it's also highly satiating, therefore keeping you fuller for longer, thereby helping reduce the chance of snacking or making bad food choices throughout the day, making it an underused tool for achieving your weight goals, regardless as to whether you are trying to lose, gain or simply maintain your weight.

Your body uses the amino acids it gets from protein to perform various processes and it can't do so effectively without them, which is why it's essential you find a way to include protein in some form at every meal. Breakfast is usually the meal that people neglect this idea the most, causing their bodies to face extended periods without protein being consumed. This becomes an even bigger issue when you take into consideration that protein intake at lunch tends to be minimal, meaning that depending on how you currently eat, your body may only be provided with an adequate amount once every 24 hours. With that in mind, this is potentially one of the biggest adjustments to work on to improve your diet. There are a variety of options available from chicken to smoked salmon or steak, as well as many inexpensive sources such as milk, cheese, Greek yoghurt, eggs and beans.

You have no doubt seen news stories about the potential health risks surrounding red meat and while in many ways they may have been misinterpreted and blown out of proportion, I still recommend leaning towards the safe side of this argument and only having it once or maybe sometimes twice a week. That way you can still enjoy red meat as part of your diet, while minimising any potential risks involved. If possible it's best to completely avoid the pre-packaged, processed meats aisle. While these products may be tempting due to their sheer convenience, most are filled with additives, preservatives and harmful chemicals, which from a health perspective, is exactly what you should be trying to move away from. Not only that, while they may appear cheaper, your money could easily be put to far better use. For example, instead of stocking up on packs of readily sliced ham for your sandwiches, you could rather buy a whole chicken and roast it in the oven. This requires absolutely minimal preparation beyond turning on the oven, putting it on a tray and cutting it up when done. A whole chicken will easily make enough meat for the week and you could apply this same principle to using a ham, turkey or any other meat you desire. If convenience really is a deciding factor in your purchasing decision, then consider opting for a rotisserie chicken or some of the other ready cooked alternatives available in most supermarkets.

Healthy options of protein include:

Meat and seafood:

- Any fish	- Chicken	- Turkey	- Beef
- Shellfish	- Duck	- Lamb	- Pork

Dairy, vegetarian, vegan and substitutes:

- Eggs	- Milk	- Beans	- Cottage cheese
- Lentils	- Soy products	- Tofu	- Greek Yoghurt

It's impossible to include everything on this list, so obviously there are other forms less commonly consumed that could be added. Don't be afraid to experiment and try other things, just use the basic principles you have learned so far to determine whether or not it's a healthy addition to your diet.

Carbohydrates

One of the main issues with the Western Diet is that foods have become heavily processed and refined, which causes the fibre, bran and various other nutrients beneficial to your health to be lost or removed. In a perfect world when choosing carbohydrates, your aim should be to focus primarily on sources rated as low to medium GI, that are unrefined, complex and high in fibre such as oats, brown rice, potatoes, or whole-wheat bread and pasta. These sources will ensure you get many of the nutrients you require, while avoiding added chemicals, sugars, and additional ingredients found in highly processed variants. Opting for these sources causes your meals to be digested more slowly, resulting in a slower, more even release of glucose into your bloodstream. In addition, complex carbohydrates keep you feeling fuller for longer and provide you with constant energy throughout the day. One of the main reasons why this is important in a balanced diet is because it helps maintain stable blood sugar levels, and doing so drastically reduces many of the health risks associated with the modern diet. This makes it an essential strategy for preventing, treating and even reversing chronic diseases such as diabetes, hypertension and heart disease, which studies directly link to continual spikes in blood sugar levels caused by high GI foods.

I however realise that this is not a perfect world, and the reality is that no matter how much I go on about why you should turn to complex carbohydrates over refined variants, you may simply refuse to do so. I have actually lost count of how many people I've spoken to who say they just don't like the taste or texture of whole-wheat or brown variants, many of whom simply flat out refuse to even consider incorporating them into their diet, regardless of how beneficial they may be. This is where so many diets go wrong, as they keep trying to force an issue that was dead in the water to begin with. Continuing to lecture people on how they have to switch to complex variants if they want to improve their diet only leads to pushing them further away from the idea of adapting to a healthier way of eating, as they are presented with an all or nothing situation, with no glimpse of an alternative insight. Not only that, but lecturing reinforces their perception that healthy eating is all about restriction, a rigid set of rules, or eating foods they don't enjoy. For this reason, it doesn't matter how 'perfect' a plan for 'optimal health' may be, it will never work if you are unable to follow it, which is why I'll be taking a very different approach in regards to how we deal with carbohydrates.

So yes, while there's no denying you would substantially benefit from making the change to low GI sources, if this is a moot point for you to begin with, then I have developed an alternative, where you can decide exactly what and how much you want to change. Having said that, if you do choose to stick to your current sources such as white bread, pasta or rice, then all I ask is that you aim to limit or reduce your intake to a few servings a week, on top of ensuring you consume sufficient amounts of vegetables. In comparison to other approaches that place them as completely off limits, I don't think a compromise of cutting down is unreasonable. If this is what you decide to do, then stick with your normal sources and judge your portion sizes in accordance to the method used in the next section, as this approach remains the same, regardless of the source from which it comes. However, I want you to aim to reduce your intake to less than five servings a week, ideally trying to keep it to around three. For other meals opt instead for healthier options such as white or sweet potatoes and for some meals, swap out the carbohydrates for two additional servings of vegetables.

The reason for this is that by including low GI foods in your meal, you lower the overall GI content, thereby reducing the negative side effects refined carbohydrates have on your body, including consequences such as rapidly spiking blood sugar levels. This is why you can still eat refined carbohydrates, but by being smarter about how you put together your meals and incorporating lower GI sources such as vegetables, you can make it far more balanced. However, don't take this to mean that just because you ate some broccoli you have free reign to eat whatever you want.

If, however you do decide to start incorporating healthier sources into the way you eat, then it doesn't mean you have to base every meal solely around them. Regardless of how healthy you aim to be, there's nothing wrong with occasionally indulging, as nothing bad is going to happen if you choose to order white pasta over whole-wheat the next time you go out for a meal. In fact, if this change is new to you, then you always have the option of using healthier variants for some meals, while sticking to what you would normally use for others. Either way, I highly advise that you try a range of different options to see what you like, without simply dismissing them as all being the same, or something you won't enjoy. I know the change in taste or texture can come as a shock, but honestly, I can't tell much of a difference and personally I actually prefer whole-wheat sources. I think for many people the problem is more mental than anything else, caused by a preconception that this is something they won't enjoy as it's different, therefore dismissing it before they even try it. So if you fall into this category, start small and work your way up. For example, if you choose rice or pasta and are anxious about making the switch from white, then initially try using half and half. You could try whole-wheat bread over white, or experiment by using other options in your favourite meals, such as lentils in your curry, or buckwheat noodles in your stir-fry.

I think it's important to reiterate the point that everyone responds differently, which is why carbohydrate use will differ from person to person. For most people it won't be a problem, but the reality is some people simply don't respond well to their consumption, in which case they may be better off on a high fat diet. It's all about listening to your body, and if you encounter any issues then you may want to substitute carbohydrates for extra servings of healthy fats, and seeing how you respond.

A different approach

I have broken carbohydrates up into three tiers and it's entirely up to you to decide which you fall into. You may even find over time that as you start eating healthier you progress from one tier to another as your palate changes and you become more open to trying new and different foods:

Tier 1: Sticking to refined carbohydrates, but limiting intake to five servings per week, with the goal of keeping it to around three. At first glance that may sound like a lot, but it quickly adds up if you have white toast in the morning, a sandwich at lunch, followed by some pasta for dinner. Which is why you should aim to spread them out across the week, and for other meals use options such as white or sweet potatoes, whole wheat bread, and swapping out carbohydrates in some meals for two additional servings of vegetables.

Tier 2: Use a mix of refined and complex sources. Whether that's using them half and half, or alternating them between meals is up to you. Make sure you don't exceed five servings of refined variants per week, and ideally aim to keep it below three.

Tier 3: Implementing a diet revolving primarily around complex and starchy sources, with a limited intake of refined sources.

I'm sure you know the various options of refined sources available, from white bread to rice or pasta, so I'm not going to fill a table with them. The options listed below are all choices that would mostly fall into tier 2 and 3.

Healthy(ier) options of carbohydrates include:

- Oats	- Brown rice	- Potatoes	- Whole-wheat pasta
- Beans	- Chickpeas	- Spelt	- Whole-wheat bread
- Rye	- Couscous	- Buckwheat	- Sweet potatoes
- Lentils	- Grain bread	- Barley	- Rice noodles
- Bran	- Quinoa		

As you can see there's a wide variety of options available to suit all tastes and preferences, from grains to pulses or legumes, giving you endless possibilities of ways to develop and incorporate them into meals. It's easy, cheap and convenient to make the switch from refined, processed variants and many of them are cooked or prepared in a similar, if not the same manner.

Fats

Due to their high calorie count in comparison to protein or carbohydrates (fats have nine calories per gram and carbohydrates and protein have four), fats are often the first thing people cut from their diet when trying to lose weight. What they don't realise though is that not only are fats extremely filling, but they are also essential for various different functions throughout your body. In fact, reducing your intake can actually be counterproductive in achieving your weight goals. It's fair to say that fats are probably feared more than any other nutrient, simply because of the wildly untrue perception that eating them causes you to gain weight. Sure, this may be the case if you consume excessive amounts, but that holds true for anything you eat. Instead, to improve your overall wellbeing, you should be looking to include healthy fats at every meal.

Omega 3 fatty acids are essential for health, yet they are largely under consumed, with large amounts of people likely to be deficient. To avoid this, you should ideally be aiming to consume fish at least twice a week, with one of those servings being from an oily source. Some of the best options include salmon, trout, sardines and mackerel. However, if you are vegetarian or don't like fish, then other options include walnuts, flaxseeds, chia seeds, various oils and soybeans.

Healthy options for fat include:

- Extra virgin olive oil
- Nuts

- Coconut oil
- Butter
- Nut butters

- Avocados
- Seeds
- Cheese

- Full fat yoghurt
- Whole eggs

Vegetables

The fact of the matter is most people don't eat anywhere near enough vegetables, with low intake levels being a huge contributor to the health epidemic we are currently facing. Reasons or excuses for avoiding them range from childhood memories to bad experiences with bland, boiled cooking, simply just not wanting to, or one of the worst objections of all, refusing to eat 'rabbit food'. Somehow many people's misperceptions lead them to automatically assume they don't like vegetables, when in many cases, they haven't even tried them. If this sounds like you, then there are a variety of ways to include them in your meals, without even realising it. For instance, you could make home-made pasta or curry sauces based around tomatoes, mushrooms, carrots, onions or spinach, try various different seasonings to change the taste on your palate, add them to your sandwiches, or even use them in smoothies. As previously mentioned, including them in breakfast can sometimes be a challenge, but you should aim to get at least two different variants added to every lunch and dinner. Ideally at least one of those should be from a green leafy option, such as spinach, kale or broccoli. You may not believe me now, but vegetables can be truly delicious and you are missing out on so many incredible tastes and flavours by excluding them from your diet.

Regardless of how you choose to consume them, to ensure all of your micronutrient needs are met, make sure you include a variety of different sources in your diet. To do this, aim to incorporate a range of different colours into your meals, as that's the easiest way to get the full spectrum of what you require.

You will no doubt have seen so far that my approach to coaching has been completely void of preaching or telling you what to do, but this is the one situation where I have no choice but to make an exception, as it simply is that important to your health. If you fall into the category of not eating enough vegetables, then there's no way around it, it is absolutely essential that you change your outlook and habits on this matter. In fact, I can't stress enough how important this really is and if you currently disregard vegetables from your diet and truly want to improve how you feel, then the first place you should focus on is increasing your intake.

Fresh fruit and vegetables are often portrayed as an essential part of a balanced diet and it's not common knowledge that in many ways, frozen ones can actually be a better option. That's because nutrients are often lost during transportation or in the time between when they are picked, packed and eaten. As they are frozen at the source, nutrients are kept intact, and this is another reason why frozen foods are often cheaper than fresh versions, as they aren't burdened by the limits of use-by dates and may be a good inclusion into your weekly food shop if you are prone to waste.

The list below contains just a few examples, but feel free to add in others you encounter. You will find various different options depending on where you live, shop or what season it is.

Healthy options of vegetables include:

- Broccoli
- Kale
- Lettuce
- Peppers
- Peas
- Beets

- Tomatoes
- Spinach
- Cauliflower
- Asparagus
- Celery
- Sprouts

- Mushrooms
- Bok Choy
- Green beans
- Courgette
- Radish

- Onions
- Watercress
- Collard greens
- Butternut squash
- Sweetcorn

Fruit

Fruit plays a vital role in a balanced diet, as it's filled with essential vitamins and minerals. It can however be high in sugar, which is why it's best to limit your intake to around two servings per day. Be that as it may, there's no cause for concern like there is over the potential health risks associated with a high sugar intake from processed or refined products. The main reason for the difference is down to fruit being high in fibre, thereby reducing the rate at which it spikes blood sugar levels. Remember that the fibre of fruits and vegetables is often located in the skin, so whenever possible, try to avoid peeling them, or you will lose many of the health benefits they offer.

Personally, I choose to have fruit with my breakfast and after exercise, but you need to find out where it best fits into the way you choose to eat. Not only is it a great post workout food, but it's also ideal as an afternoon snack, a healthy after dinner alternative to chocolate pudding, or whenever you want something sweet. It's best to avoid dried fruits though, as they can often be filled with added sugars and preservatives, making them far from the healthy snack they are perceived to be. The same goes for tinned fruit, as often they can come packed with syrups and additional preservatives. This however is not always the case, so make sure you read the packaging to get a better idea of exactly what you are consuming. Just like with vegetables, if you are worried about waste, frozen fruit is an ideal choice and can easily be used in anything from smoothies to desserts or in meals.

Again this is a non-exhaustive list and I highly recommend you try a range of fruits. There are so many incredible options out there, all of which can introduce a whole new world of flavours, tastes and textures into your meals.

Healthy options of fruit include:

- Bananas	- Apples	- Oranges	- Strawberries
- Papaya	- Grapefruit	- Cherries	- Pineapple
- Limes	- Peaches	- Any melon	- Raspberries
- Kiwi	- Blueberries	- Lemons	- Other berries
- Grapes	- Plums	- Mangos	

Flavourings

One way to make your meals not only taste great, but include further nutrients is by using various herbs, spices and other flavourings. The items listed below are widely used in cuisines around the world and have a host of health benefits from cancer-fighting properties to anti-oxidants, vitamins and minerals. Trying new flavours is a great way to make meals more interesting and add variety to your diet. Simply adding one to a regular meal can completely change the way it smells, tastes and feels, which can be an essential strategy if you easily get bored with what you eat.

These flavourings will have little to no effect on your overall calorie intake, but could have a huge impact on how you enjoy your meals. Because of that, feel free to include as many of them as you want. Depending on your culture, where you are located or what cuisines you enjoy, there is a whole host of different options available, meaning its worth having a look at what else you can find.

Some ideas for flavourings include:

- All herbs	- Garlic	- Ginger	- Chilli
- Salt	- Pepper	- Turmeric	- Paprika
- Lemon juice	- Lime juice	- Cinnamon	- Soy sauce

In supermarkets you will also find seasonings with many of these flavourings mixed together, with just some examples including garlic pepper, BBQ, piri piri, fajita mix etc.

Other factors to think about

By now you should have a good idea as to whether or not something is good or bad for you, and while I do keep reinforcing the notion that nothing is restricted, you still need to focus on limiting or controlling your intake of foods that are less beneficial to your health. Every decision you make has the ability to either nourish your body, or fill it with toxins, and while making bad decisions can move you further away from your goals, at times they are simply necessary for peace of mind. Sometimes you just need to give in and enjoy yourself and there's nothing wrong with occasionally doing so. At the end of the day, what you eat is one of the few things in life you have complete control over and by finally accepting this, you can break away and be free from the control food has over you. That's why I said to follow the general rule of aiming to consume around 80 to 90 percent of your calories from whole, unprocessed sources like the ones listed above, with the rest of your intake being made up of whatever you desire.

Improving the way you eat

"Once you have to start counting calories, it takes away from the joy of eating."

- Mireille Guiliano

Portion sizes

Whether you are looking to lose, gain or just maintain your weight, getting the correct sized portions will be an essential factor in determining your success. This is one of the reasons why people are put off by the idea of healthy eating, as they have the misperception that eating this way involves the tedious task of counting and tracking every single calorie consumed. This practice is however both unnecessary as well as impractical, and for many people can actually be bad for their health, as all it does is further push them towards obsessing over what they eat and spurs on problematic relationships with food.

There's no denying that we have got used to consuming ridiculous-sized portions and this in turn has had an undeniable impact in contributing to the soaring rates of obesity. There have been countless studies on this issue and the reoccurring trend in findings is that the larger the portions of food dished up, the more likely it is you will overeat. This has come to be known as a 'mindless margin', as it's very easy to either over or under eat, without even realising it. To give you an example of how big an issue this can be, let's say on average you burn roughly 2,000 calories a day, meaning that's the amount you would need to eat in order to maintain your weight. Now let's say you overeat by 10 percent everyday (which is around 200 calories). While that may not sound like much, in reality that equates to around 20 pounds of weight gain across the year and chances are you wouldn't have felt like you were overeating at all. That is why changing the way in which your meals are served is such a key factor in making this change.

The good news is that the opposite is true as well, and by reducing portions to a more sensible amount, you will consume fewer calories. Not only that, but once you understand how to control your portion sizes and develop an awareness for how much you eat and how much your body burns, controlling your body weight will come with ease. Portion control is about far more than simply eating less and if anything, understanding the differences between the foods and drinks you consume, along with knowing how to adjust your intake accordingly is far more important.

From a mindset point of view, it's been proven that we naturally want to eat roughly the same amount of food each day, which is why restrictive diets are so challenging and leave you with such a tremendous appetite. The way around this is to satisfy your desire for food volume and controlling calories by increasing portion sizes of some items, while reducing the size of others. In essence what it comes down to is practicing calorie control by making smart substitutions, thereby removing the need to starve yourself. By filling your plate with high fibre, high water, low calorie foods such as vegetables and limiting the amount of space taken up by higher calorie options will allow you to actually consume more. On top of that, these substitutions are far more filling, in turn playing a big role in helping you deal with hunger or cravings.

How to put this into practice

Regardless of your goals, portion control is going to be a vital strategy due to the fact that it directly influences the outcome you desire. That doesn't however mean you have to go breaking out the food scales or counting every grain of rice, as luckily there is a proven method widely used around the world to determine how much you should be eating. The best part is it can be done anywhere and anytime, without the need for any fancy equipment.

You probably haven't realised this, but your hands are proportionate to your body and because of that, you can use them as a tool to measure out how much of each nutrient you require.

With that in mind, a serving of protein should be around the size, thickness and diameter of the palm of your hand. Fats (such as oils, nuts, butter) should be the size of your thumb (or half of say, an avocado or one egg), and carbohydrates and vegetables the size of your fist each. A portion of fruit is roughly the equivalent to half a large fruit, one medium-sized fruit, two smaller ones, or a fist sized portion of items such as grapes.

How many servings of each nutrient you need varies depending on your individual circumstances, such as your goals and how you eat your meals. For instance, eating more regularly and having four to six meals a day will determine that you break servings up into smaller portions when compared to being split over three meals. Just like everything else, there is no one-size-fits-all correct model to determine the amount you need and finding out what works for you will require a trial and error process to see how your body responds.

For a reference point though, the average woman's daily requirement will be between three to six servings of each nutrient, which is about one every meal. Men on the other hand require nearly double that amount, needing around six to eight servings per day, or roughly two for every meal.

How you break them up depends on your personal eating preferences and the foods you choose to consume. Regardless of how you do it, just make sure you get at least five servings of fruits and vegetables everyday.

To put this in perspective, if an individual ate three balanced meals a day then:

An average meal for women would be:
- (1) palm-sized portion of protein
- (1) fist-sized portion of carbohydrates
- (2) fist-sized servings of vegetables
- (1) thumb sized serving of fat

An average meal for men would be:
- (2) palm-sized portions of protein
- (2) fist-sized portions of carbohydrates
- (2) fist-sized servings of vegetables
- (2) thumb-sized servings of fat

If you find after meals that you are still hungry, then add an extra portion or two of vegetables. Since they are low in calories and high in fibre, they will help fill you up without drastically increasing your calorie intake or negatively affecting your weight goals. Additionally, if you are following tier 1 and dropping refined carbohydrates from a few of your meals, then add in a couple of servings of vegetables to increase the volume and you can do this in the other tiers as well if you are making a largely vegetable based dish. If you think outside the box, there are some great healthy ways to put together meals, for example: you can make cauliflower rice by dicing it up in a blender or cutting courgettes into strands, making it similar to spaghetti. Don't feel like this approach means that you have to stick to two vegetables at every meal and can't swap them out for other forms. For instance, if you like variety and are making something like a salad or pasta sauce, then feel free to reduce your vegetable portions to half a fist-size or smaller.

Meal ideas

With all the ingredients listed, there really is no limit to the options available for what you can choose to make. Below are just some examples of meals you could prepare using the principles above of selecting an ingredient from each of the categories.

Breakfast

- Oats, banana, peanut butter, Greek yoghurt and cinnamon
- Poached egg and avocado on whole wheat toast
- Tomato, mushroom and onion omelette, with garlic and chives
- Buckwheat pancakes with banana, egg, cinnamon and Greek yoghurt

Lunch

- Grilled paprika chicken, with tomato, avocado and spinach on whole meal bread
- Tuna salad with tomatoes, mushrooms, sweetcorn and olive oil
- Jacket potato, with cheese and beans
- Lentils and chickpea stew with pine nuts, peas and carrots
- Grilled chicken with sweet potato fries, broccoli, green beans and olive oil

Dinner

- King prawn spaghetti with tomato, broccoli, mushrooms, garlic and olive oil
- Grilled salmon with asparagus, baby potatoes and butter
- Chicken stir fry with buckwheat noodles, broccoli, pineapple, beansprouts, soy sauce, chilli flakes and coconut oil
- Lentils curry with brown rice, peas, onions, tomatoes, turmeric and coconut oil
- Beef stew with new potatoes, broccoli, carrots, brown rice and olive oil
- Garlic lemon butter prawns with baby tomatoes, spring onions, parsley and rice
- Steak with mashed potato, butter, peas and mushrooms
- Grilled cod with, garlic lemon butter sauce, homemade chips and peas

Eating in regards to your weight goals

Obviously, the amounts discussed above will vary depending on your size, goals, activity levels and how many meals you decide to eat per day, but they are a good general guideline to use as a starting point when determining what you actually need. Just remember that wherever possible, you should be aiming to consume some form of each nutrient at every meal, as this is the only way to ensure your diet is balanced.

In order to determine how to eat for your weight goals, try to adapt to this way of eating, with the aim of consuming roughly the same sized portions everyday and track your weight changes for two weeks. You should be looking to do so in as similar conditions as possible to limit the possibility that results are influenced or affected by a change in circumstances. So select a day to weigh yourself where you will be able to do so on roughly the same time and day, use the same scale and do so wearing the same, similar, or no clothes, preferably first thing when you wake up after going to the bathroom.

Depending on what you eat, it's common for excess water to be stored by your body, and this can fluctuate massively depending on higher intakes of carbohydrates, salt or sugar. This excess water is often referred to as 'water weight', and it tends to quickly be lost when calories are reduced. It's for this reason that many diets can claim miracle fast results, especially in cases where they remove carbohydrates, when in reality, those results are merely lost water and not fat. Depending on how much is stored, you can easily see one to two kilos lost within the first week or two, which is why you won't be looking to make any changes within this initial period. If after two weeks your weight remains the same, then you will have a rough idea of the amount of food required for your maintenance level, which simply means the amount you need to consume for your weight to stay the same. Whereas if you are gaining weight, you know you are eating too much, and if you are losing weight, then you are consuming less than you require. Once you know this, you will be able to adapt your calorie intake accordingly depending on the results you desire.

From then on you can continue to track your weight if desired, again doing so on the same day and under the same conditions each week until you reach you desired weight. After that you can just eat at maintenance level, aiming to consume roughly the same amount of calories each day, and without worrying or overthinking as to whether you have gone slightly over or under.

What changes in weight should you be aiming for?

Remember, this way of eating is all about sustainable change, and because of that, your goal shouldn't be drastic weight loss or gain. Instead, you should be aiming to lose weight at a safe rate, which is around one to two pounds per week, or 0.2 to 0.5kg. I know that doesn't sound like much and isn't the quick turnaround you are probably hoping for, but anything more drastic than that will result in a high amount of muscle mass lost, in addition to slowing down your metabolism. Meaning that as and when you return your eating patterns to normal, chances are you will quickly regain the weight that was lost. On the other hand, while this approach may take longer, it has the added benefit of the weight actually staying off. It's important to note however that individuals with more weight will initially see higher levels of weight loss, but they will eventually average out to more moderate amounts.

With that in mind, once you have used this approach for the first couple of weeks and evaluated your progress you may need to either increase or reduce your calorie intake in order to get your weight goals on track. Doing so can either be done by increasing carbohydrate or fat intake, however you will need to make a judgement call on how much to do this by, as it will very much be based on just how far off your loss or gain was from your target.

If you do have a weight target, then track your weight weekly, because as you move closer towards your goal, it's inevitable that in time, weight loss or gain will slow or potentially even stall. If this happens, then after a couple of weeks men can either add or remove one fist-sized serving of carbohydrates to a meal of their choice, or one thumb of fat, and women can remove half that amount. At the end of the next week revaluate and repeat if necessary, until you find the amount needed to maintain your current weight, or are once again seeing a safe level of either weight loss or gain.

Please note; it's common for weight to fluctuate daily depending on what you eat or the amount of water your body stores. I have even noticed up to a kilogram difference from day-to-day measurements, which gives you a good indication of how much it can be impacted. This is why I want you to wait two weeks before reducing or increasing your intake, to enable you to see if there really wasn't a change, or if the reading was simply influenced by another factor that day. This is why you should always aim to track your progress at the same times and in similar conditions, in order to limit the possibility of the readings being influenced.

I can't reiterate enough that the entire purpose of these changes is to develop a lasting, maintainable, healthy lifestyle, with losing weight as an added benefit, not the primary focus. That's what sets this apart from other programmes, and it's because of that if your weight doesn't change as expected one week, that it's vital you don't get deterred or beat yourself up about it. The reality is you will have good and bad weeks and regardless of the reasons why, obsessively monitoring and fixating on weight loss will only place added pressure on yourself mentally, which in turn will further drain and challenge you emotionally. With how stressful everyday life already is, this is added pressure you simply don't need and is one of the many reasons why the majority people fail to ever make any lasting change. So who cares whether it takes six weeks or a year to reach your goal. All that matters is that not only do you get there, but you stay there as well. That's why instead I want you to focus on enjoying the journey and your newfound better health for what it is, not just obsessing over the outcome.

"You 'can' be in control. And I stress this, because there's so many things going on in my life that I'm not in control of. And that's my message. You can control your outcome of your body. Eat to live, and don't live to eat."

- Evelyn Oswick

How often should you be eating?

One of the major problems with misconceptions about health, nutrition and fitness is that in theory they often seem to make perfect sense, making them easy to buy into and believe. In turn this can make it difficult to change our beliefs, or accept someone else's idea if they dispute the misconception we believe to be true. In part this helps explain why people are so set in their ways, as well as why they can be so defensive about their habits and behaviours.

One of the biggest myths I bought into for a long period of time was that eating small meals more frequently causes your metabolism to keep continuously working throughout the day. The idea behind this is that nutrients are more effectively put to use, thereby resulting in increased fat loss over the course of the day. This is the reason why the fitness industry's standard advice is to eat small meals every few hours, and people are continually told this is the optimal strategy to burn fat and lose weight. In theory it makes perfect sense and while it is true your metabolism goes up when you eat, studies prove the amount it increases relates directly to the proportion of food consumed. This is more commonly known as the 'thermic' effect of food and the net effect is the same whether you spread the food out over three meals or six.

In direct relation to this, another widely believed misconception is that regular intake of food stops you from overeating and curbs your hunger. Again, in theory it makes perfect sense. You are giving your body a constant supply of fuel to top up its energy levels, which would prevent feelings of hunger. However, it took me a long time to realise that in fact, doing this was having the exact opposite effect on my satiety. By having smaller meals, I was never satisfied and even before finishing a meal I was immediately thinking about the next. I was never comfortably full and this got to the extent where I spent everyday counting down the three hours until I could next eat, causing me to fixate over the thought of food. A mindset that in hindsight was both unhealthy and filled with negativity. I started to contemplate the idea that something was wrong with me. Perhaps my metabolism was messed up, or maybe I had some sort of imbalance in my diet since I was always hungry. I changed up what carbohydrates I ate, tried different fats, added more vegetables, yet still, I could never shake the constant feeling of hunger. At one point I even 'self-diagnosed' and convinced myself that maybe I had diabetes, as that was the only thing I could think of to explain how I felt.

It wasn't until the holidays when I had some time off work and was at home eating three large meals a day that I actually felt normal and realised the error of my ways. By eating larger, more filling meals, I was finally giving my body enough food to be satisfied. Not stuffed, but comfortably satisfied. For the first time in a long time, food was no longer on my mind and I could go hours without obsessing over when my next meal was coming. Eating this way gave me a sense of freedom and a clearer mindset, I had increased concentration and contrary to what I previously believed, I had more energy. Furthermore, I also reduced the stress I was directly placing on myself by never being able to shake the desire to eat from my mind, as before I faced a daily battle struggling with hunger and cravings, combined with the irritability and on-edge feelings that comes with it. I found that when eating regular, smaller meals I had daily periods where I felt off, slightly lightheaded, dizzy and drained. In fact, come 3pm and it was simply an expected part of my day and it was only by eating that I could temporarily feel normal again. I have found from my own experiences and the people I have worked with that it's actually during this time that you are more likely to binge or overeat. This is down to simply wanting to shake those negative feelings and emotions, as often you will turn to any glimpse of hope in doing so.

Taking a different approach

Most diet plans range from suggesting you eat three meals per day, with two snacks in-between, to eating six to eight smaller meals every couple of hours. We have already established though that most diets don't work, so contrary to what's popular and because of the reasons discussed, I'm going to recommend that instead, you try just eating three larger, more satiating and balanced meals, with no other direct snacking or grazing throughout the day.

For some of you the idea of changing up your eating like this may come as a shock, as you are left thinking that by doing this you will have to face struggling with cravings and hunger all day. I know that's the conclusion I would have jumped to if it had been suggested to me, as that's exactly why I ate the way that I did for so long. However, when I incorporated eating three big, balanced meals into my lifestyle on a daily basis, I found the exact opposite to be true. This approach drastically changed the way I thought and felt, which is why if you are hesitant or pessimistic about changing your behaviours, then all I ask is that you take a leap of faith in trusting me with this one and giving it a go. While initially it was strange not to be eating every few hours, after a few days I actually preferred the bigger meals and it was a huge relief mentally to no longer have food constantly on my mind. I easily settled into the new routine without any hassle or struggle and it quickly became a new and lasting habit. Eating like this has helped many people I have worked with lose weight easily and effortlessly, simply through the knock-on effect of removing the constant internal battle of dealing with willpower and obsessing over food, therefore directly improving their overall mindset and happiness. Furthermore, having three larger meals requires less meal preparation and planning, giving you more time to live your life.

There is however an exception to this and that's for people who are highly active or regularly engaging in exercise. That's because depending on where it fits into their schedule, it may require adding an additional pre or post workout meal. Personally while I aim to have three larger meals a day, on days I work out it's usually increased to four.

But it's your journey

As with everything else, everyone responds differently, and because of that, it's all about finding out what works best for you.

Therefore, while I do think this change in approach will benefit most people, I also recognise the fact that it may not suit everyone. So if eating three meals and a couple of snacks a day is what you enjoy doing and fits into your lifestyle, then by all means continue to do so, especially if those snacks consist of fruits or vegetables and are helping you increase your overall micronutrient intake. Ultimately this new lifestyle is all about finding ways for you to be healthier in a maintainable way, not trying to force you into something you can't stick to, or simply don't like doing. However, before you dismiss the idea of changing your habits, take some time to have an honest reflection as to whether or not you only eat the way you do because that's what you are used to, as chances are it's merely down to routine and the habits you have formed. If you find yourself regularly snacking or grazing and turning to foods that negatively affect your health and are constantly facing challenges to your willpower, you could have a much easier time transitioning into a healthier lifestyle by changing to only three meals a day. In fact, from a weight loss perspective probably the biggest advantage of eating in this manner is that it stops you from snacking, which usually tends to be on high calorie foods that are causing havoc with your progress.

After a lifetime of eating the way you do, it's natural to be pessimistic or doubtful about this change, and if this is the case for you and you can resonate with the examples that I have shared, then I highly recommend that you at least just give it a try for a couple of weeks. During that time you can see how your body responds, giving you a true indicator as to which approach is best for you.

"It's not the plan that's important, it's the planning"
- Dr. Gramme Edwards

Strategies for getting round the barrier of time

Improving the way that you eat will in many ways come down to one single factor – proper planning. That's why when life's hectic and you are in a rush, it's all about making the healthy option the 'easy' option, as by thinking ahead about what you are likely to be consuming, you will be able to get a better idea of how to fit healthy meals you enjoy into your routine. The way I have made this work for me is by creating a range of quick and easy-to-make meals to eat during the week. I have three different breakfasts I can rotate between and on Sunday afternoons and I tend to bulk cook my lunches for the week so that they are all prepared ahead of time. It means eating similar foods, but at least preparing them like this gives me complete control over what goes into them and drastically cuts down on time spent cooking. I make sure they are all dishes I enjoy, so I don't mind the repetitiveness and can even leave adding spices or flavourings to the very end, meaning I can actually make them all taste very different. Besides, I can always change them on a weekly basis if I want to.

Eating similar foods for breakfast and lunch isn't as bad when you vary your evening meals and although it may sound like a drag, if you think about it, many people tend to eat similar, if not the same foods for breakfast and lunch anyway. As far as evening meals go, I have a range of dishes made from ingredients that go well together, but taste vastly different depending on the type of dish I'm preparing. Using similar ingredients and planning ahead reduces and streamlines the thought process, so although the basic premise remains the same, the protein, carbohydrates, fats and vegetables are all interchangeable, meaning I can adapt it depending on what I feel like and therefore don't have to follow a rigid, set out meal plan.

To give you an example of this, I could get home in the evening and decide to make a pasta dish using chicken, tomatoes, broccoli and mushrooms. I could just as easily replace the pasta with rice or potatoes and use different spices to make a curry or stir-fry, meaning that my ingredient combinations are incredibly easy to customise, allowing my palate to enjoy an array of tastes with minimum effort. What this has done is put the healthy option on autopilot, as it has just become something I do without having to stress over or think about.

Eating this way saves money on grocery bills, as I know exactly how much of everything I need every week, making my amount of waste pretty much non-existent. With some planning I have managed to reduce my shopping trips to once a week, which again saves time and effort. While it takes some initial thought, once you have figured out how and what you like to eat, the process is actually a straight forward experience. I find my evening meals only take around 15 to 30 minutes to prepare, and I have several options that can be thrown together in under five minutes if I'm tired, in a hurry, or really don't feel like cooking. Meaning it's hardly much of an inconvenience compared to that four-minute micro meal or takeaway, but with all the added benefit of being nutritious and tasting better.

Once you have got rough idea of how you aim to eat, you can use this knowledge in conjunction with the strategies listed below:

Make a meal plan

Chances are you will eat at least some of the same foods on a regular basis, which is why I highly advise you sit down and make a meal plan for the week ahead. That way you know what most meals are likely to consist of, making it less likely you will act on impulse and turn to other convenience offerings instead. This is probably the biggest issue of them all, as it's been found that it's during these moments that we are more likely to make negative choices, such as turning to takeaways or other processed foods. This is a great way to get the whole family involved, and I have found doing so has the added benefit of making kids far more likely to be accepting of a healthier way of eating, as they feel like they have an input and this 'change' isn't being forced upon them.

Depending on your individual circumstances, you can even take planning to the point where you decide which member of your household is responsible for cooking on particular days, lifting some pressure off your shoulders and allowing family members to explore their inner chefs! Initially it's best to keep things simple and start with seven days at a time, but as you get more comfortable, you could easily extend your planning further.

Make a weekly shopping list

Shopping can be an inconvenient and time consuming experience, but by having a list for your meal plan you can save a massive amount of time in store, as you won't be aimlessly wandering around trying to decide what you need.

Shop online

You could even take this a step further and use a home delivery service. Once set up you can quickly add regular items to your list, reducing your weekly shop time down to a matter of minutes. Many stores now have apps you can quickly and easily use to complete your weekly shop and in most cases you pay exactly the same as you would in-store.

Bulk cook

Find a day or afternoon where you can free up some time and prepare as many meals as possible then freeze them. The extra effort involved for making larger portions is minimal and can save you a huge amount of time in the long run. By having a freezer stocked with healthy nutritious meals, you can quickly throw one in the oven or microwave after a long day, removing the temptation of turning to take away on nights that you are too tired to cook. You could even pack and prepare a few days lunches ahead of time, meaning it's no longer a daily chore on your to do list. This method also has another advantage that is often overlooked, which is the fact that it reduces your gas and electricity bill.

Make extra for lunch

If you are eating out for lunch most days you will probably be struggling to find healthy options. If you don't feel like preparing lunch, then just make a larger dinner and take left overs with you the next day.

Make extra and freeze it

If bulk cooking doesn't appeal to you or you don't want to eat the same meal two days in a row, try cooking larger dinners and freezing the leftovers so they are there for another day.

Turn to other healthy convenience foods

On days you really don't feel like cooking, instead of turning to takeaways, get a rotisserie chicken or other ready-made freshly prepared items. Not only are they fresh and delicious, but they are free from all the chemicals and processed ingredients you should be aiming to avoid and you can quickly prepare a salad, some vegetables, rice or anything else you would like to go with it.

Prep ingredients when you get home from store

If you are rushed for time in the evenings, try chopping up vegetables or other items when you get home from the store. Keep them in Tupperwares ready for use, and you can quickly throw together anything from a stir fry to a pasta dish or salad in under 15 minutes.

Keep fridge stocked with precooked proteins

Roast a chicken or other meat on a Sunday, chop it up and store it in the fridge ready for use. It will last for up to four days, meaning it massively cuts down on preparation and cooking time, in addition to being a go-to protein source for your meals.

Set up cues

Try setting up cues that encourage you to act upon healthy actions. For instance, if you regularly skip breakfast, one thing you can do is to place everything you need out on the counter the night before. This will act as a visual reminder of what you need to do, thereby making it less likely you will skip it. An example of this in action is by having everything ready for you when you get up, you can quickly throw some oats in the microwave, slice some banana while they are cooking, then add some peanut butter and Greek yoghurt. There you have a filling nutritious breakfast, prepared and eaten in under ten minutes.

Strategies for eating socially

Regardless of who you are or how much you are looking to change, it's inevitable that certain challenges will get in your way. For many people the biggest hurdle is trying to do it surrounded by family and friends who aren't embarking on the same journey, which in turn can often place them in situations filled with temptation. Whether they are work related, family gatherings or just catching up with friends, social situations always tend to be the hardest to keep control of. A small treat can quickly turn into an all-out binge, which is why as hard as it may be, you need to learn to be mindful of your actions and focus on your behaviours. I'm not saying don't enjoy yourself, but just be wary that it's easy to undo a whole week's worth of hard work and perseverance in one nights eating or drinking.

That's why it's essential you explain to friends and family why this is so important to you, and get them to realise you need help and support, not to pressure you to 'give in just this once'. Peer pressure to them may seem harmless, such as 'don't make me drink alone', or 'one slice of cake won't make any difference', but those instances can often lead you off course. This is especially true during the initial stages of change, where you are more likely to be adapting or struggling with making better choices, making it harder to not give in. There are however various strategies you can apply to these situations, and you will find that implementing them can go a long way in not hindering your progress.

Strategies for eating socially include:

- If eating out, plan ahead by looking at menus beforehand. Most restaurants share their menus online so you shouldn't have an issue finding them. That way you can determine the healthiest options in advance and won't feel under pressure to decide in the moment.

- On days you know you will be going out or indulging in the evening, have a lower calorie lunch like a salad and opt for a high protein breakfast.

- When in a self-service or "all you can eat" situation, impose a rule where you only allow yourself to go for one serving and if you are still hungry, only go back for additional salad, fruit or vegetables.

- Eat a small filling meal such as some Greek yoghurt and drink one to two glasses of water shortly before the meal. This will help partially fill you up, making you less likely to overeat.

- When indulging in excessive amounts of food, try and limit your alcohol intake.

- If you are having dessert, opt for fresh fruit.

- Wherever possible, avoid foods that are deep fried, battered or breaded. Instead go for something that has ideally been grilled, sautéed, steamed, baked or roasted.

- If you are unsure how a certain dish is prepared or what it contains don't be afraid to ask.

- You can make substitutions by asking to swap your fries for a salad or vegetables. That way you regulate calories, while still enjoying the main part of the meal.

- Be mindful about your decisions. Do you want more because

you are hungry? Or simply because there's food available on demand?

- Avoid 'super sizing' when eating fast food.
- Opt for two starters instead of a main meal at a restaurant.
- If eating out, avoid ordering any additional sides.

With all things considered, it's important to remember that food from restaurants is full of added salt, sugar and fat, making it near impossible to judge how many calories you consume. Therefore, the only way to have more control over what goes into your food is to eat out less. That doesn't mean you should avoid social situations and stop living life, but far too many people use food as entertainment, which is a behavior and habit that is highly detrimental to their health. If you find yourself regularly in these situations, then try and find ways in which you can change them. For instance, suggest doing social gatherings at home where you can have control over the food prepared, rather than eating out.

Strategies to help with portion control and snacking

If you are used to eating excessively large portions, then getting used to practicing proper portion control will be a vital part of your success. I know it takes some getting used to, but below are some tactics you can use to make it easier:

- Put down your fork or spoon in between bites and chew slowly. This forces you to slow down how quickly you eat, allowing you to savour each mouthful and in turn making it far easier to start recognising when you are full.
- Use smaller plates and utensils. This will help you control the amount you dish up and consume in each bite, having the knock-on effect of your brain estimating a larger volume of food, due to the plate being smaller.
- Never eat or snack directly from the package, as it makes it harder to keep track of how much you have eaten. Instead determine how much you will be having and serve it on a plate.
- Pre-portion snacks and treats into smaller bags.
- Pre-serve items such as protein and sides in the kitchen, then keep salads or vegetables on the table in easy reach. That way you if you are tempted by seconds you will be more likely to choose them over the higher calorie alternatives.
- Pre-measure your portion in advance and pack away any leftovers for the next day, so you can't go for seconds.
- It takes 20 minutes for your brain to recognise you are full, so if you are still hungry after a meal, drink a glass of water and wait 30 minutes before deciding if you want more. The reason for

the water is to make sure you aren't mistaking hunger for thirst, along with cleansing your palette. This is because we often want more of something if we have a lingering taste in our mouth, so removing it may get rid of the craving.

- Again as it takes time to recognise when you are full, if you are trying to lose weight, then eat slowly until you feel you are 80 percent full.

- Have a high fibre breakfast that keeps you full until lunch.

- Keep a bowl of fruit on your kitchen counter, as you are more likely to go for healthy snacks if they are readily available and in sight.

- Studies have found that you are three times more likely to choose to eat the first thing you see than the fifth, so don't keep unhealthy foods in sight or at the front of your cupboard.

"Strength does not come from physical capacity. It comes from an indomitable will."

- Mahatma Gandhi

Willpower and cravings

When looking for ways to explain bad decisions or reasons why they gave in to temptation, a lack of willpower is usually people's go to response for what to blame or use to justify their actions. The reality is that no matter how strong you are, everyone only has a finite amount of willpower, and because of that the more often it has to be exercised, the harder it becomes to resist. This is often why when you are continually challenged throughout the day, it gets more difficult to endure. In fact, one interesting study on the matter found that when queuing in a coffee shop it's easy to say no to the first few cakes and pastries you see. But by the time you reach the till, every item you have seen has tested your willpower, making it far more likely that you finally cave in if you are offered anything else. Researchers suggested this is not only because of the drain on your willpower, but also because you subconsciously think about how good you have been recently with saying no to everything else, therefore making you deserving of a treat.

Although you can improve the strength of your willpower, the main problem is it simply doesn't work in relation to addiction, and while you may think strong willpower is an essential trait to have when eating healthier, studies have found your food environment is actually a significantly bigger factor in determining your success. This is because changing habits takes time and until your new practices become part of your everyday routine, it's far easier to reduce temptation by changing what's in your kitchen and the way you eat, than it is to constantly have to try and remain strong in the face of adversity. I have found personally that the best strategy to improve your willpower is to find ways to change your environment, as doing so will limit how often your willpower needs to be used, and avoid it being tested. You can do this by removing the temptation, along with visual cues and reminders, as this eases the amount of strain you place on yourself, making it easier to resist. The aim is to create a situation where you would have to go out of your way to give in to sweets or food, and this could involve anything from removing all junk food from your house, to changing where you have lunch. You can even leave your wallet at home so you can't take any action when tempted by an afternoon snack. You just need to find out where, when and what challenges you face, so that you can find ways to lower the impact or exposure you have to them. Over the next few pages I will be giving you some ideas that have worked for either me or people I have worked with, but it will be up to you to decide which actions you incorporate in your daily routine to help you.

For instance; many people tend to snack when they are bored, due to the temporary comfort and relief given by high sugar, fatty or salty products. By ensuring you only have healthy options in the house, will make it more likely that you will only eat if you are hungry. After all, turning to munching on carrots when you are bored is not an urge many of us have, whereas a bag of cookies is a completely different story. This is why I stopped stocking my cupboards with foods like chocolate, cookies and other items that fall into the category of 'junk', as by removing the temptation, it limits the times I choose to indulge. Obviously, at times you will still get cravings, but the age-old saying of 'out of sight, out of mind' is especially true in these circumstances. Not only that, but you will find that as you start eating healthier, your cravings become far less common. By not having them on hand, you remove the instant gratification option, which means you can't simply give in on impulse, making it much easier to make the right decisions. I know this action is far from easy, especially if you live in a household with others who aren't embarking on the same journey. In this case, it may be a wise idea to try and get the whole family involved with improving their health, finding ways to compromise and change their behaviours at the same time.

Other strategies to help deal with cravings and willpower include:

- Tell yourself you have to wait 20 minutes before deciding whether or not you will give in to temptation. Cravings are usually temporary, so by stopping yourself from acting on impulse you give them a chance to pass and this is a vital strategy for improving your willpower.

- Decide you can have what you are craving, but you have to wait until tomorrow to do so. Then see if you still want it just as much then. Chances are the feelings will have passed, as you will have had time to re-evaluate what you want and what's more important to you. Then if you still decide to have that treat, you can do so knowing you waited and truly it, which in turn will help strengthen your resolve.

- Drink a glass of water or tea, as cravings for sweetness may in fact be an indication that you are dehydrated.

- If it has been over three hours since you last ate, try having a healthy meal to see if the feelings weren't just being caused by hunger.

- Think about your frame of mind. Are the cravings a result of stress? Are you anxious or in a situation that causes you to seek comfort? Try the breathing exercises mentioned earlier in this book or remove yourself from the situation by going for a walk. Alternatively, you could call a friend, go for a run, read a book, listen to music, or even just vacuum the house.

- If you keep getting cravings for sugar, try eating something else sweet instead, like fruit. Not only is this the perfect way to satisfy your desire for sugar, but it also increases your micronutrient intake, and if you are trying to change your bad habits, could be the perfect replacement for that afternoon snack.

- Find ways to make healthier versions of the foods you are craving so that you can satisfy them guilt-free, or at least reduce the negative effects that they have.

- Make sure you are getting enough sleep. Studies have found a lack of rest can cause you to crave carbohydrates and sugar due to the short-term bursts of energy they provide. In fact, in 2012 the Mayo Clinic even found that people who slept 80 minutes less than they normally did ate 550 calories more than usual the next day.

We have placed a large amount of focus so far on finding ways to streamline processes and make things easier, so if willpower is something you really struggle with, probably the best strategy is to plan ahead and shop online. Not only is it more convenient, but it removes the risk of impulse buys, taking away in-the-moment decisions, as you no longer face the rows of chocolates and treats tempting you while you are waiting in line or browsing through the aisles. Studies have found that as much as 80 percent of candy and 61 percent of salty-snacks are impulse purchases, which just goes to show how influential product display can be. So by removing yourself from the situation, you remove any chance of being led astray.

Shopping can often be a stressful experience, especially when you are in a rush, tired or hungry. Unsurprisingly, studies have shown that when in this frame of mind, you are more likely to make bad decisions, as outside influences tempt your already stretched willpower, causing you to seek a quick release of comfort offered by many of the products you are trying to cut down on. For that reason, if you don't want to or can't shop online, then at the very least, eat before you shop, and make sure you have a planned list of exactly what you need. Likewise, try sticking to the outer isles where the fresh products are located, and avoid going into any areas that force you to test your resolve.

'Treat' meals

One of the best ways to help with your willpower is to plan a meal every week or two where you indulge in something you otherwise wouldn't as part of your new healthy lifestyle. Be that a Friday night take away, Sunday afternoon lunch, going for ice cream, or any other occasion that appeals to you. In most diets these are often referred to as 'cheat' meals', which in this regard is a phrasing that I am really against. All this term does is fuel negative relationships with food, by portraying these items as something you shouldn't be having, and placing them on a pedestal out of reach. From this point forward you are no longer dieting and because of that your new way of eating is not something you can 'cheat' on. Instead all you are doing is ensuring you have a balance of everything in what you consume, which includes the occasional 'treat' meal. This meal does however give you something to look forward to, which can really help in times when you are challenged by temptation. The more you practice this outlook, the easier resisting at other times becomes. It's important though that you don't view this meal as something you earned through good behaviour by resisting on other occasions, as a huge part of developing a healthy relationship with food is breaking the cycle of using food as a reward. It's essential that when you do choose to indulge that you don't go overboard, as it's not a license giving you free reign to binge. You need to learn to savour these meals for what they are, which is why you need to keep them to one meal, and not a whole day.

Approaching healthy eating with the mindset that nothing is restricted or off limits helps massively with reducing the mental strain most diets tend to cause. Not only that, but it gives you a sense of accomplishment that you have control over your emotions, rather than them controlling you. What you may even find after a period of eating wholefoods and finding ways to make healthy versions of your favourite meals, is that your desire to indulge drastically decreases along with your cravings. In fact, you may even come to resent how awful you feel afterwards. That's one of the main reasons why I very rarely eat fast food. Not just because it's bad for me, but because I hate that sluggish, uncomfortable feeling afterwards, where your stomach feels off, followed by that sugar crash shortly after, and it's even worse when sometimes that feeling last for a few days.

Moderation

I know I have said the best approach is to remove temptation, but in time you may get to the point where you are able to practice proper moderation with what you consume. What this means is being able to have appropriate portions, and be satisfied with doing so, as you are able to appreciate foods for what they are. This way of thinking is a mindset that many people are able to reach, allowing them to have a truly balanced and varied diet.

On the other side of this though is the unfortunate reality that for some people moderation simply does not work. I'll no doubt be criticised heavily for saying so, as it's contrary to what most other health writers will say, but it's something I have come to accept as true. Personally moderation is a part of my mindset that I have always struggled with and no matter what I do or try, it's an aspect I simply can't get fully under control. The truth is I'm a classic binge eater. I can't have just one biscuit or block of chocolate, because as soon as I start, I just want more, and it always ends being the entire pack. That's why personally I would rather have nothing, than put myself though the anguish of the cravings and willpower battle that follows after having a small amount. I would love to be able to tell you there are methods or strategies everyone can use to change this (and for most people there are), but the reality is this is just how some of us are.

But does that mean you need to live a life of depriving yourself of the foods you love?

Definitely not. That's why I spent so much time finding healthy alternatives and learning the best ways to prepare them. That way I can still enjoy anything from burgers to pizza and a range of desserts, so I never have that feeling I'm missing out. Best of all, they aren't packed full of sugar or processed ingredients, and I genuinely mean it when I say that I have actually come to prefer these healthier options. Sure, I still occasionally treat myself. But when I do, I approach it in a similar manner as to how you don't enter a casino with more than you can afford to lose. What I mean by this is that I only buy what I don't mind finishing, and I only do it on certain occasions. Approaching it in that manner saves the feelings of guilt, as at those times I have made a conscious decision before hand on what I choose to enjoy, meaning I can do so without any feelings of regret. This is not however an approach that is necessary for most people, as by being mindful in the practice of taking smaller portions and savouring them, the skill of moderation can be developed.

We all react and respond differently, which is why for some things you simply have to make a choice between what you want now and what you want most. It's all about finding out what you are capable of and able to do, listening to your body, and doing what feels right for the lifestyle and mindset you desire.

"No one is born a great cook, one learns by doing."
- Julia Child

The importance of cooking

In order to truly eat healthier, I think one of the key issues and biggest changes that needs to be made is finding ways of incorporating more cooking into your lifestyle. Doing so is the only way to get complete control over what you put into your body, making it an essential strategy in achieving a balanced diet and avoiding deficiencies. Far too many people are put off by the idea of cooking, perceiving it as something they don't know how or are unable to do. This is often due to the misconception that it's complicated, stressful or takes hours, which is the last thing anyone would want to do after a long day at work. But in my experience the 'I don't know how' excuse mostly just means they simply don't want to, and the only way to change this mindset is to find meals that are not only quick, easy and convenient to make, but also delicious. The reality is cooking is far from the overwhelming experience it's perceived to be and you can make it as simple or as complicated as you desire. I'm far from a chef and everything I have learned has been through starting with basic meals and making small adjustments to them in order to try new things. By doing so I turned the daunting prospect of being in the kitchen to a passion I now look forward to and enjoy, giving me an outlet for my creativity, on top of helping me relax and unwind.

If you are not already doing so, then I highly recommend giving cooking a go and if you are, then it can't hurt to try and make some more time for it. The only way to get better is by taking some basic recipes, along with some ingredients you know you like and trying different things with them. That's how you learn, and how you find ways to create a diet that revolves around great tasting food you love and look forward to eating. If you can get really good at making a few recipes, cooking becomes quick and hassle free, even when you are exhausted and by regularly practicing and doing it everyday, it simply becomes part of your routine. You will naturally head to the kitchen when you get in from work, rather than reaching for the packaged alternative, and you will prefer the outcome produced by those few extra minutes of your time. At first meal preparation may feel slow and tedious, but once you learn what you are doing, it becomes quick and easy. Like with everything else, it just takes practice. As we discussed earlier, by having a plan or strategy for your approach you can enjoy the process rather than trying to work it out as you go. Be that as it may, don't feel like you need to be restricted in what you do, as one of the most rewarding actions in cooking is simply going with it and seeing what you create.

"Beware of little expenses; a small leak will sink a great ship."
- Benjamin Franklin

Eating healthy on a budget

There seems to be a huge misperception that healthy eating is an expensive luxury, and this is frequently used to justify poor diets, food choices and purchases. While it's true that healthy food can cost more, with a little thought you can easily eat well on any budget. The problem is people just don't seem to know how to do it, regularly blowing their hard earned cash on a range of unnecessary products, that often just go to waste. There's no denying our society wastes far too much food, with the average UK household throwing away around six meals per week and American households disposing of up to 50 percent of what they buy! Waste isn't just limited to those countries either, as approximately half of the world's food is going to waste every year!

When it comes to food, the issue of heath and budget stretches to another level. The idea of "convenience" plays a massive role in how we choose to consume our food, often meaning that healthy food is the first compromise to be made, in favour of a quick and cheap meal. For example, KFC constantly promotes the concept of their 'value' family buckets being a cheap alternative to cooking, since you can quickly feed the entire family without much expense. Instead you could buy a whole chicken at a supermarket, along with some potatoes and vegetables. Since you probably didn't feel like cooking in the first place, how about you buy a rotisserie chicken instead like I suggested earlier in the book? Both your bucket and your chicken can feed a family of four with minimal effort, but the second is done without all the harmful additives, extras, and ridiculous amount of processed oils, with the added bonus of being cheaper in most cases as well.

That's just one example of this being put into practice, but with some careful consideration, there's a whole host of other ideas you can use.

Strategies to reduce your food bill

Remember how we explored some strategies for making sure you have time to cook? Most of those will automatically also reduce your food bill as well!

Plan meals

One of the easiest ways to reduce your food bill and eliminate waste is to plan your meals for the week ahead of time. This prevents you from having to decide what to have on a whim, and makes it less likely you will turn to eating out.

Make a shopping list

Linking directly to planning meals, this involves making a list for the week of what you need and implementing a rule where you only buy what you are sure you will use. This takes some practice to judge and get right, but I have now reached the point where my food waste is pretty much non-existent. The Journal of Nutrition Education and Behavior found that shoppers who had written grocery lists purchased healthier foods, and it was deemed this was down to them being less likely to make impulse buys, which usually tend to be spur of the moment decisions for products you don't need.

Shop online

If you struggle sticking to your list or being distracted by impulse purchases, then the easiest way to avoid this is to shop online.

Cook at home

Those takeaways and restaurant dinners add up to far more than you think, especially when done regularly, in fact, research has shown that the average British person spends over £4000 on dining out each year and the average American spends $232 per month! That's why the easiest way to reduce your costs is to eat out less. Even if you land up spending extra at the supermarket, you are spending money on your health, adding in nutritious ingredients and bulking your meals with healthy options!

Pack lunch

In the moment buying lunch may not seem like a huge cost, but over the course of a week or a month it quickly adds up. Buying your typical sandwich, drink and snack deal averages around £3.50 a day, which based on a typical 48-week work year adds up to £840 year. You could easily at least halve that amount by making your own lunch.

Opt for single ingredient whole foods

Make sure you go for products with as little additional processing as possible. For instance, readily grated cheese or vegetables that come ready cut cost substantially more than they do in their original form, with it being common place for some to cost over four times as much!

Stop purchasing 'junk' foods

You would be amazed at how much you could save by reducing purchases of empty calorie items that offer no nutritional value, such as sodas or sweets. This is one of the biggest gripes I have with people who moan about healthy eating being too expensive, as a floret of broccoli is about one-fourth of the cost of a two-litre soft drink bottle, which many families drink several of a week.

Look for sales to stock up your cupboards and freezer

If it's something you eat regularly and has a long shelf life, then take advantage of opportunities to stock up your pantry whenever you can. Be careful though, as this can easily go both ways, encouraging you to buy excessive amounts of products you don't need, which you are then forced to either eat in excess, throw away, or get stored in the back of a cupboard, never to be seen again.

Check the going out of date sections

As products start nearing their sell by dates supermarkets drastically reduce their price in order to get rid of them as quickly as possible. Don't let this put you off though, as there is often quite a big difference between the sell by and use by date, meaning there's absolutely nothing wrong with using these items. When they are discounted varies from store to store, but if you time it right you can make huge savings on everything from fresh meat to seafood, fruits, vegetables, or a whole host of other products. Try shopping at the end of the day or first thing in the morning to take full advantage of these offers.

Go meatless for some meals

I know, the thought alone may sound like a nightmare, but believe it or not you can make some delicious meat free alternatives of your favourite meals. Try using other protein sources such as eggs, canned fish or legumes. Personally this was a concept I was really sceptical of at first, but in reality after a few meals I barely noticed the change, especially after finding a way to make a delicious chickpea, lentil and bean curry.

Buy produce that is in season

Fruits and vegetables that are in season are far cheaper, as they are more readily available and don't need to be imported.

Go frozen

If you are prone to throwing away fresh produce, then the easiest way around this is to buy frozen variants instead. Similarly, if you realise halfway through the week that you have items such as fresh fruits, vegetables or herbs that are likely to go off, make sure you freeze them before it's too late.

Buy in bulk

For items such as oats, rice, pasta and other dried or canned goods you can get huge discounts at wholesalers or distributors by purchasing in bulk. They also have a long shelf life, meaning they aren't going to go off in your cupboards. Just make sure that you only buy larger quantities of foods you actually eat, and aren't simply buying them for the sake of thinking you are saving money.

Try cheaper, unbranded goods

Everyone knows branded goods cost more than supermarket's own unbranded alternatives, but what we don't realise is that in many cases, they offer no improvement on taste or nutritional value. Yet we buy them simply due to the mindset that a fancier label must make them better.

Look for coupons

Check your local supermarkets website before shopping to see if there are any offers or promotions. These may be included in local papers or magazines, so check before throwing out any junk mail. If you choose to shop online there tend to be monthly offers and promotions on various different sites, meaning it pays to spend some time looking around.

Check your cupboards

We are all guilty of losing track of what's lurking in the back of our cupboards, so when planning your meals double check what you actually have. Not only could this save you from buying duplicates of products you already have, but you may get some inspiration for other meals you could prepare from what's already there.

Grow your own

While not feasible for everyone, if you have the space you could easily plant a small vegetable garden that requires a minimal amount of maintenance. Doing so will not only save you money, but may be a relaxing and rewarding activity, which tastes better than the store bought alternatives. I tend to mostly do this for herbs, which over the course of the year saves a substantial amount.

Final thoughts

As you can see, eating healthy is definitely a viable option for everyone, regardless of their budget and these are just a few of the ideas you can take and apply to your circumstances. Reducing your food bill is a relatively simple action to achieve, but it may just require you to think creatively or make some changes to the way you approach your meals and embrace change. Essentially what it all comes down to is properly evaluating your current decisions and behaviours, then planning ahead to ensure you can take more positive actions in the future.

Putting it all together

"One of the best pieces of advice I ever got was from a horse master. He told me to go slow to go fast. I think that applies to everything in life. We live as though there aren't enough hours in the day, but if we do each thing calmly and carefully, we will get it done quicker and with much less stress."

- Viggo Mortensen

I said in the introduction that it was my goal for this book to be different, so hopefully now you can see that the long-winded approach to get to this point was designed in a way of taking you down a path of self-realisation. I really wanted you to think about the bigger picture, as you break away from traditional approaches and shift your focus from being all about eating less and moving more, to instead finding a balance that is maintainable long-term. There really is more to our wellbeing than meets the eye, which is why we took a holistic approach to ensure you fully comprehend what's involved, along with the true risks and repercussions of failing to act upon it. The reality is you are far more likely to make sustainable change if it's not only something you want, but also something you truly believe in, which is hopefully the state of mind you find yourself in now. When you get right down to it, motivation to do something often has little to do with the task itself, and instead is based on how you view it. By changing your perceptions and how you think, will have enabled you to view this process in a whole new light, allowing you to recognise the true benefits of pursuing this course of action.

Many of the latest fitness and 'healthy eating' trends fail so spectacularly, as they are mostly based around external motivations, which in the long run, are rarely reason enough to keep you going. In the grand scheme of things external motivation basically makes dieting seem like punishment for overeating, or exercise as a prescription for weight loss, thereby forcing you into actions you don't want to take. On average, we only last around 19 days following a diet, before giving up and resuming our old routines, which is evidence in itself that we need to do this differently.

That's why so much time was spent looking at what constitutes towards a healthy lifestyle, as it was my intention to change the way you view and approach everything from food to your mindset, activity and rest, consequently enabling you to shift your hope for change, to a desire for action, and later on, to the lasting result you wanted. This was all done to help you find your internal motivation, which is an essential part of this process. By shifting your thoughts to what you have to gain and why you are doing it, rather than what you are giving up, you will make the entire process far easier and more enjoyable. So stop thinking about external factors like society's perceptions of what it means to look good or be healthy, and instead focus on eating foods that help you thrive, becoming more active and finding inner clarity and acceptance, along with happiness and longevity for you and your family.

I hope you enjoyed all of the content covered so far, and it opened your eyes to the actions that are negatively influencing your wellbeing on one hand, all while opening a whole new world full of health and prosperity on the other. You now have all the knowledge you need to make more informed decisions, and as a bonus, you also know far more about health, nutrition and fitness than the majority of people. Now it's time to put everything you have learned together, as you start your journey to take back your health and become the best version of yourself.

So what next?

By this point you are no doubt eager to begin, but I would like to reiterate that going forward is all about slow, gradual change. Yes, I know that goes against your basic instinct of wanting to do everything right this instant, but trust me and try it my way, regardless of any doubts or reservations you may have, as this is the best way to make change that is maintainable long-term.

"A goal without a plan is just a wish."

- Antoine de Saint-Exupéry

The 3P's - Plan, Practice, Perfect

Your success in achieving goals in any area will very much come down to what I like to call the 3P's – plan, practice, perfect. These are the basic principles I coach my clients on when developing new habits, and will be the basis of the approach we use going forward.

You are going to be making roughly two changes every two weeks, one in your diet, and one in another area of your lifestyle. I know that doesn't sound like much, but if you think about it properly, in three month's time that will be roughly 12 changes you have made that not only have a resounding impact on your wellbeing, but have also become a part of who you are.

With that being said though, this process is all about you and the changes you want to make, which is why this pace is very much a guideline for the path you will be taking. You may find that as you progress, in some weeks you will be able to focus on a couple of smaller habits, whereas larger changes may require more attention and take longer. There may be times when life gets in the way and you have pull it right back, or you may even find some habits and actions intertwined, helping you progress at a faster rate. Just always remember, developing new habits takes time, so if initially new actions don't feel as automatic as you hope, then don't feel discouraged, as you will get there. I just want you to take it as it comes, without placing any additional pressure on yourself to try and force it to happen. Ultimately as this is such a tailored approach, it will very much be a trial and error process, as you learn to adapt and adjust accordingly as you go.

In order for this process to work I want you to accept right here and now that there will be times when you will slip up or backtrack. You will mess up and you won't always get it right or see the progress you expected. There will be good days and bad days, times you smash your goals and times you need to take a step back to indulge and enjoy life. What you need to keep remembering is that the goal is progress, not perfection. That's why above all else, consistency is key. You need to be aware of the choices you make, and try to make the right decision as often as you can, without dwelling on the times you don't. That's what will allow you to truly keep moving forward.

However, just because I don't want you to stress about it, doesn't mean you can be completely laid back about the entire process and brush it all off. It's still going to take hard work, dedication and commitment, where you actively need to push yourself in order to achieve your goals. Just like with your diet, many things in life are about the 90/10 rule, where you should be aiming to make the decision that's best for your health most of the time, and not stress over the times you choose to enjoy yourself.

So what now?

At the beginning of this book I got you to start getting into the habit of practicing working on small changes, with the goal of adding more vegetables and fruits to what you eat, drinking more water and actively finding ways to walk more on a daily basis. This was all done to get you used to focusing on and practicing the implementation of small, healthier habits everyday, in addition to building a foundation on which to grow, mentally preparing you for what's to follow. These actions are however vital for your health's longevity, so I want you to ensure that you continue to practice them from here on out. Now it's time to add to them further, focusing on changes that are personal to you.

In order to complete the tasks over the next few pages, you will need a few pieces of paper and preferably a couple of different coloured pens, along with your food diary and the list of goals you made earlier in this book. If you struggle to free up time, you can always tackle the habits and food planning separately, but please complete them as near a time to each other as possible.

"Life's challenges are not supposed to paralyze you, they're supposed to help you discover who you are."

- Bernice Johnson Reagon

Improving your diet

For many people whose eating habits revolve mainly around processed foods, the move towards a diet based primarily around wholefoods can initially be a difficult transition to make. So while the end goal of having a diet largely consisting of foods from natural sources is a good target to aspire to, as with everything else, it's essential you don't try to do too much too soon, or overhaul everything at once. That's why we are going to start by focusing on improving one meal at a time, practicing it until you get it right, and only then moving onto the next. To do so I want you to use the methods covered in the how to put together a balanced diet section, in conjunction with applying these principles to creating meals.

It has been found that when asked about our eating behaviours, we tend to unintentionally exaggerate good choices and underestimate bad ones. This is often done subconsciously to justify to ourselves decisions we know we shouldn't be making, or simply because the instances we indulge are down to habits or in the spur of the moment, therefore being forgotten about altogether. That's why in an earlier section I got you to keep a food diary for a week to keep track of what you were eating, ensuring that you ate in exactly the same way as you normally would. Doing so will allow you to get a complete overview of your actual decisions, routines, habits and actions, together with finding patterns and cues that may explain both the causation and temptation leading to negative behaviours.

Look back at it now. Does anything surprise you? Do you remember the moment you ate everything listed?

Chances are you have never really paid much attention to what you were actually eating in the past, which is why another purpose of this task was to get you to be more mindful about what you are actually consuming. This will go a long way in developing healthier habits, as by recognising your behaviours you will mentally start to question when and why you make detrimental decisions in the future. This in itself can go a long way in improving willpower, getting you to more consciously think about your actions, how often they are occurring, and if they are truly something you want.

Evaluating your food diary

Ideally, map out your food diary on paper or print it off so you have it out in front of you. This will be the best way to get a bird's eye view and compare your actions on a day-to-day basis. Then, using a different colour pen, highlight and make some brief notes next to the areas you recognise are causing the most harm. Underline instances where you have gone massively off track and look for trends in eating patterns, situations that lead you astray and regular actions you can link to everyday habits and routines.

Once you have done that look for meals containing highly refined or processed items where you could include more fruits and vegetables, or switch to a healthier option instead. For instance, changing to whole-wheat bread for your sandwiches, or replacing that sugary cereal for oatmeal. When all is said and done, we are creatures of habit, which is why you will more likely than not start to notice similarities in your behaviour, so it should be pretty clear to see where you might be going wrong.

Moving forward

Step 1:

Now that you have a better idea of how you have eaten over the course of the week, it's time to use your findings to make a list of all the aspects negatively influencing your health that could be improved. It's absolutely essential to be brutally honest with yourself here, as this is not the time for excuses or justifications. Instead, it's all about self-reflection and using this as an opportunity to get a better idea of why you behave the way you do, along with why you need to change or potentially cut back on the amount of instances you choose to indulge.

For example, some questions you could ask yourself or instances you could highlight may include: do you always make bad choices when going out for lunch? Or, do you always have something sweet after meals? Maybe every afternoon you have a cup of tea and some biscuits? Do you turn to a sugary snack to get through the midday slump? Do you skip breakfast? Do you head straight to the pastry section when getting your morning cup of coffee? Are your lunches always void of any vegetables?

Take as long as you need to thoroughly think this through, as the more thought and detail you put into it, the better.

Step 2:

Next, think about how you feel when you eat. Do you stop when full, or do you always finish everything on your plate? Are you eating because you are hungry, tired, stressed or lonely? Do you always eat while watching TV? Or maybe you always get a takeaway every weekend?

By recognising and understanding the areas in which you make bad decisions, you can work out where you need to consciously focus on improving. Not only that, but you can also get a better understanding as to whether or not your food related behaviours are linked to your emotions or environment.

Make sure you keep the list, as we will be coming back to it shortly, as answers to these questions will help in the next section when determining what habits you need to change.

Step 3: Focusing on one meal

For the first part of this process, I want you to focus on one meal, making it as healthy as possible, as regularly as you can, before moving onto the next meal. From my experience, two weeks tends to be the perfect amount of time to get it right, especially when you actively look to make smaller, more informed decisions in other areas of your diet at the same time. Working in this manner will allow you to get used to the changes, without the feeling of giving up foods you are used to or love, as you aren't trying to overhaul your entire diet at once.

The most important factor here is to be consistent, so make sure you try and practice this new habit each and everyday, until it becomes something you no longer have to force or think about.

How you are going to do it

Step 4: Meal one

Your first point of call will be to start with the meal you feel you have the most control over, is likely to be the easiest to change and to which you can dedicate sufficient time to practice. This will vary from person to person, but for most, breakfast is probably the best option to start with. That's because it tends to be the meal people are the least fussy about, as well as being the easiest to prepare and get right. Furthermore, it has the added benefit of beginning your day with positive change, which can have a resounding effect on your mindset for the rest of the day, directly spilling over into your success in other areas. If you currently don't eat or regularly skip breakfast, this could be a great time to start finding ways to incorporate it into your daily routine, and if need be you could even prepare something to eat during your commute, or even at your desk with your morning cup of coffee.

Practicing this habit may require getting up slightly earlier, but in order to make this process as simple as possible, try to plan and prepare whatever you can ahead of time. What you choose to eat will determine whether you should put out the ingredients ready for use in the morning, or even cooking the night before. Planning ahead will mean you can make your decisions on what to eat when you aren't under the pressure of time, hungry or feeling lazy, thereby making it far more likely you will make positive choices.

If you are short on time, you could even try some other recipes such as overnight oats or chia seed puddings, or even some baked breakfast muffins or quiches. Other options include scrambled eggs on whole-wheat toast, or if you have a bit more time and want to add more vegetables into your diet, you could even chop your vegetables the night before and the next day make an omelette filled with tomatoes, onions, peppers and mushrooms. Obviously these are just a few ideas, and depending on your routine and dietary preferences there will be a variety of options available for you. Whatever you do though, just aim to move away from the usual high sugar cereals and breakfast bars often turned to when in a rush and aim to ensure you find a balanced meal that incorporates protein, healthy fats and slow release complex carbohydrates.

Step 5: Meal two

Once you are used to having breakfast, you can move on to trying to prepare and pack a healthy lunch to cut back on trips to the canteen, deli or fast food options. Initially this may take some extra effort, which is why proper planning is once again, the key. That's why it's best to aim to do this the night before, as that way you can avoid having to rush around in the morning. Whether you want to bulk cook on weekends, make extra for dinner so you have leftovers, or prepare something entirely different, is up to you. Again, I want you to practice this for two weeks, ideally each and everyday, while still ensuring you maintain your new habit of breakfast.

I know lunch may be slightly more challenging, especially in our ever busy world of working lunches, networking events and other occasions. If that's the circumstances you find yourself in and it's simply unfeasible to practice this habit everyday, then there are other measures you can look to follow that will keep you on track. For instance, if you are regularly going out to restaurants you could look at menus beforehand to get an idea of what's on offer and what the healthiest option would be. At the same time, you could change your fries for a side of vegetables, or ensure that regardless of what you order, you get a side salad as well. Or even better, order a starter with a salad to cut down on the excessive calories often found in main courses. On the other hand, if you find yourself in a self-service buffet situation, then make sure that at least half your plate is filled with salad, fruit or vegetables. Set yourself a rule that you won't go back for seconds, and ideally avoid the dessert table, since let's be honest, the options they have on hand are normally pretty bland and really not worth the calories they contain, meaning you are far better off saving your treats and indulgences for items you actually enjoy. This in turn will help in breaking the habit of simply consuming these items because they are there, helping you move away from making decisions purely based around in the moment satisfaction.

Step 6: Meal three

Dinner is usually the time when you can incorporate the most variety into what you eat, get your creativity going and find ways to build meals around the foods you love. This action may require pushing your comfort zones, getting yourself to start spending some time in the kitchen and experimenting as you go. However, if cooking is new to you, then it may be best to initially stick to simple and easy to make meals that you are sure you can get right. Doing so will help boost your confidence, get you into the habit of cooking, and ensure you are creating balanced meals, without the added pressure and frustration of trying something new when tired after a long day. Then on weekends or days off when you have more time, you can try new recipes and look to further add to your meal plans. Again, planning and thinking ahead will be absolutely essential, as it will be all about making the healthy option the easy option in a way that works for you, while trying to avoid the mindset of just wanting to eat and get it over with.

Step 7: Snacking

By actively making more informed choices, chances are this will have influenced the way you snack. However, if this is yet to have happened, then once you are in the routine of having three healthy meals a day, then your next step will be improving your snacks. This may involve replacing that afternoon chocolate bar with some fruit, other healthy alternatives such as a pot of Greek Yoghurt or even baking your own goods. The possibilities for healthy, nutritious snacks are endless, but ideally aim for whole, single sourced foods such as fruits, vegetables or forms of protein wherever possible. If however you opt for something else, then at the very least check the ingredients list on the back of whatever you choose. Your main goal in this regard is to cut down on as much added sugar as possible, as snacking tends to be a key area in people's diets where things go wrong.

Bonus

If you want to take this a step further, then I highly recommend you move towards the habit of only eating three larger meals a day, with no snacks in-between. I discussed the reasons behind doing so earlier in the 'how often should you be eating' section, and this is a habit I highly recommend you at least try pursuing. This change could be hugely beneficial if you are someone who regularly deals with obsessing over or thinking about food, or constantly have the urge to snack, as it will go a long way in improving your behaviours and mindset, along with your willpower, cravings and relationships with food.

Other considerations

The process outlined above is very much a blueprint for your success, but depending on your preferences, schedule or routine, it may not be the ideal approach for you to take. So feel free to change the order in which you approach focusing on improving meals, as in all honestly, it really doesn't matter which one you work on first. I have simply suggested breakfast as that tends to be the starting point that works best for most people. If for instance you work nights, have other commitments that disrupt regular patterns, or simply want to start somewhere else, then there's nothing wrong with focusing on lunch or dinner first, then building on it from there. Just make sure you choose the meal that you are most likely to get right, as initially it's all about succeeding in developing new habits.

While at first I'm only getting you to focus on one meal at a time, that doesn't mean you can completely disregard everything else you eat during the day. Even though that one meal is where you are placing most of your focus, I still want you to make sure that no matter what, you have at least five portions of fruit and vegetables, along with aiming to make healthier choices whenever you can. All positive actions will aid in getting you into the mindset of making better overall decisions, which in turn will play a huge role in your progress.

Just remember though, the goal is not to be perfect or eat right 100 percent of the time. That simply isn't feasible or sustainable long term. Instead, you should be trying to ensure that 80 to 90 percent of your intake is in line with fuelling your body with the nutrients it requires, with the rest free to consume whatever you desire.

Summary

To recap what you will be aiming to do:

Week 1

Focus on having a healthy breakfast everyday, and actively try to make better decisions with whatever else you choose to consume. On top of that, ensure that you eat at least five portions of fruit and vegetables.

Week 3

Introduce having a healthy lunch everyday, while still ensuring you continue to practice the habit of having breakfast.

Week 5

By now, having breakfast should be a part of your routine that you either no longer have to think about it, or are actively doing everyday without much resistance. So along with focusing on lunch, it's now time to improve dinner.

Week 7

Now that you have changed your intake for your three main meals, it's time to see what other areas still have room for improvement and to start making better choices in regards to snacks or treats.

Anything else?

As you progress with these changes, it's worth repeating the activity of making a food diary after six weeks, but feel free to do it at an earlier date if you desire. That way you can see how your behaviours have changed, and highlight areas in which there is still room for improvement. This will help you clarify as to whether or not there is enough balance in your diet, along with being a useful tool in determining if you are getting the full range of nutrients you require, and not accidentally missing anything out. You can then use this information as your focus point in week seven onwards. In fact, you could benefit from repeating this activity on a regular basis, as doing so will continually reinforce the mental aspect of being mindful about your behaviours, and you could do so until you reach a point where you feel comfortable with your eating choices and habits.

"If you are facing a new challenge or being asked to do something that you have never done before don't be afraid to step out. You have more capability than you think you do but you will never see it unless you place a demand on yourself for more."

- Joyce Meyer

Creating new habits

Now that we have covered how to improve your diet and implemented a plan for how to do so, it's time to move your attention over to improving other aspects of your wellbeing. The only way to alter behaviours is to acknowledge their existence, find the triggers and rewards encouraging them, accept the reasons why they happen, why you want to change them and actively work on reacting differently. Behaviours form through continual repetition, as your mind associates certain situations and actions with how you respond to them. Therefore, by being aware and mindful about situations and decisions that negatively affect your health, you can change your responses and consciously make better choices until they become ingrained within you, taking the place of the detrimental behaviours that were there before.

You will find many programmes designed around changing habits that map out exactly what they want you to work on and what they want you to do. They dictate everything from what and how to eat, to when to wake up and exercise. This inflexible approach is far too generic, and the failure to target or consider the personal situation of the individual flaws the very foundations on which they are built. That's why I spent so much time developing the approach featured within this book, testing it with people from a range of backgrounds, with varying goals, circumstances and beliefs. All done to ensure the methods laid out can be applied and made a success.

I meant it when I said I wanted to do something different, that actually works and gives you the results you desire, which is why I based my thinking all around the help and support I wish I had when I started my journey. With that in mind, going forward probably won't be what you expect and the methods used will take some work on your behalf. On that account getting started with this approach does take some time, thought and consideration. That's the only way we can ensure that the changes you make are about you, your goals, wants, needs, circumstances and lifestyle, as well as being maintainable long-term. Before continuing you should make sure you have an adequate amount of time to dedicate to completing the following tasks, as it will take around 30 to 60 minutes to complete.

To help make the planning and layout of this process easier I have put together various activity sheets you can print off and use.

These are available at: **www.tailoredlifestyles.co.uk/activities**

"Planning is bringing the future into the present so that you can do something about it now."

- Alan Lakein

Becoming a better you

To complete the following process, firstly read through the step so that you know what's involved, think about it for a moment, then read it again before working on the activity discussed within it. Then when you are done, continue onto the next step. I want you to approach it in this manner, as doing so will allow you to apply your full focus and attention to each part as it comes, without thinking ahead about what's to follow.

Before we begin, I want you to remember how important it is that you think about how you can make positive changes in more than one area of your wellbeing. You should not be ignoring your mindset, the way you eat, becoming more active, or getting more rest and recovery, regardless of what your personal goal is.

Step 1:

Earlier in this book I got you to think about and start listing several goals you would like to achieve. Since then you have worked your way through a host of new material, covering a range of issues that you may have been unfamiliar with before, let alone considered as playing a role in your health or as something you would like to achieve. So before moving on to step 2, I want you to take a moment to reflect on your initial thoughts.

Think about your goals again, adding to or amending your list of what does being fit and healthy mean to you? What is it you want to do? And what do you want to achieve?

After everything we have covered you may find that your initial thoughts, outlook, opinion and goals may have changed. That's why I got you to do this at the start, so that you could see if the self-realisation aspect of this book altered the way you think or view what you want to get out of this process. You may however find that they are still similar, or even the same. There's no right or wrong response, but it's essential to think about, as doing so will either reinforce your initial desires, or get you started on a completely different path.

Step 2:

Now in a separate list, think about the reasons and motivations for why you want to do this. Is it for your family? Lower your risk of disease? Improve your health? Enable yourself to start engaging in more activities and experiences where your health previously held you back?

Too often people will simply state their motivation is to lose weight, but this is far too simplistic of a reason and is never the full picture. So if that was your initial thought, then I want you to think about why you actually want to lose weight. Most than likely there will be an underlying reason, such as wanting to ensure you improve your health so you are still around in 20 years for your kids. Really think about why, deep down inside, you truly want to change. Everyone's internal motivation is different. But by working out what yours is and writing it down, you will have something to refer back to every time things start to get hard and you need a little extra push, or you simply want a feel good reminder of why you started. You may even find you have more than one thing that motivates you, which is great. That means you have multiple reasons to help keep you committed.

Step 3:

For this step you are going to be using your two lists, along with the one you made on your eating habits and food diary. I want you to take into consideration what you have learned about yourself regarding your behaviours and your habits, and compare where you are against where you would like to be. To do so, use the 'Step 3' activity sheet from the download pack at www.tailoredlifestyles.co.uk/activities.

Alternatively, you can divide a piece of paper into four squares, naming each one with a different area of your wellbeing. Ensure you give each aspect the attention it requires, as the last thing you want, is to make the mistake of simply focusing on diet or exercise, and overlook the other two.

What I want you to do is to thoroughly think about each of the pillars of your health and what changes you would like to make in order to improve that aspect of your wellbeing. It's essential you are honest with yourself here, as the answers you give will form the foundation on which your healthier lifestyle is built and the way in which you develop solutions to these problems. Don't worry about the length of the list you come up with either, as the longer it is, the more you have to work with. If it's too small you have probably not taken into consideration all the pillars.

In order help you make this list, you could ask yourself some the following questions, then write the responses down under the heading for each section:

- What behaviours or factors are negatively affecting your health?
- What's stopping or holding you back from changing?
- What do you want to achieve?

As an example of this, let's consider the fitness pillar and what potentially your responses may be:

- Getting in home from work tired and not having the motivation to exercise.
- Always driving to avoid having to walk.
- Not sure what you should be doing in the gym.
- Would like to build up to doing a 5k charity run next year.
- No one else in the family is active difficult trying to do it on your own.
- An ever changing work schedule making it difficult to plan for regular workouts.
- Would like to be able to walk up the stairs or to the shops without getting out of breath.
- Lack of activity has led to substantial weight gain and would like to lose 50 pounds.

The purpose of these questions is to give you an opportunity to honestly reflect on your current health and lifestyle, all while giving you a list to work on, that's a mix of what you would like to achieve, changes you recognise you need to make, and areas you are already trying to address, but could do with more attention.

When considering current behaviours, try to look for patterns between your actions and causation, cues that lead to regular bad choices, or correlations between how one action leads to another. Your food diary is a useful tool for this, as you can use it to work out if there are any relationships that exist between certain situations and the food choices you make. For instance, those biscuits with your afternoon cup of coffee, or the trip to the vending machine after a stressful meeting. You can also consider other factors, such as struggling to find motivation to exercise after a long commute, or having so much to do in the evening that you can never find any time for yourself to just relax.

By recognising both your bad habits and the barriers affecting your progress, you can think of ways to replace them with positive actions or limit their effect. For example, if your commute home is what's causing your lack of motivation to exercise, then you could look for ways to either go straight from work, fit it in at lunch, or even do something when you wake up. Alternatively, if you have too much to do in the evening, you could potentially find ways to streamline processes, such as bulk cook dinners on weekends, or recognising you spend too much time checking emails and social media at night, which is time you could use to focus on yourself instead.

Step 4:

Now it's time to look at what actions to set to help you achieve your goals, as these will form the basis for the habit changes you will be implementing. So take your list, and as you go through it point-by-point, think of an action you would need to take in order to achieve each point, and write these out on a separate piece of paper. It's important to be as specific as possible, as while an overall objective of 'exercise more' is good, it's not measurable and there's no accountability to hold you to do it. Instead, aim for something like 'go for a 30 minute run every Monday, Wednesday and Friday'. This is much more specific, in addition to giving you a target and schedule to adhere to.

An example of this could be: if your goal is to improve your mood, energy levels and outlook on life, doing so would in all likelihood require that you make sure there's no deficiencies in your diet, and therefore the action that would need to be taken is to ensure you consume at least five portions of vegetables and fruit everyday. You may also need to address the amount of stress you are under at work, meaning it may be a case of finding ways to relax or unwind in the evening, attending a class, or changing your evening routine so that you can catch up on sleep.

Part of this this step involves breaking long-term goals into short-term targets. This is essential as not only are short-term targets easier to achieve, but they are also easier to resume if you temporarily get off track. The reality is no matter what happens there will be setbacks, which is why you can use this as an opportunity to revise goals you feel you are unable to do. By making your goals smaller, it reduces the risk that you will become disheartened or want to give up during difficult times. For instance, while there is nothing wrong with having an overall target of say 'losing 20 pounds', that in itself is a pretty daunting and overwhelming prospect, where a lack of progress could quickly discourage you. Therefore, simplifying it to 'lose a pound a week', makes it far more manageable. Not only that, but it structures it in a way that allows you to track your progress, so you can see if you meet your target each week.

Another reason for having smaller steps is that achieving goals and reaching targets gives you a feeling of accomplishment. This spurs you on to keep going as you progress and makes it easier for continual evaluation as you go. Like with anything else, what you initially perceive to be the correct way of doing something may change over time as you try new things. In many cases, it may even be a trial and error process that evolves as you go. However, while it's good to simplify matters, your new habits need to be challenging enough to keep you interested, which eliminates the risk of you getting bored or dismissive of the ideas. It's important to remember that as you progress your goals and desires may change, so feel free to continually update or add to the list whenever you feel necessary.

Regardless as to whether your decisions are based around nutrition, fitness or other changes in your life, it's essential that the goals you set are realistic. For instance, taking the previously mentioned goal of losing 20 pounds and saying you want to do it in a month isn't viable, realistic or even safe. Consequently, a goal like that would just set you up for failure and disappointment. In this case, the one-pound-a-week example is perfect, as it's specific, realistic, achievable and maintainable, while also featuring a timeframe you can monitor and adhere to. In addition, it helps control setbacks, as some weeks you may only lose half a pound, and while you didn't fully meet the target, there's still a feeling of achievement. On the other side of this, the implications of an unrealistic goal can bring on doubt or loss of motivation, as you start to question whether or not you can actually do it.

While weight loss may be a huge factor in motivating you to change, you will be far better off concentrating on goals related to your overall wellbeing that don't cause you to obsess over food or body image. By focusing on your overall health, you can make more long-term sustainable progress, with weight loss being an added by-product of these changes, rather than a short term fix. For instance, eating more fruit and vegetables, walking more, along with drinking more water are habits essential for improving your wellbeing, but chances are they will also directly lead to weight loss. Therefore, you will have a far better time mentally focusing on finding ways to increase your intake, rather than stressing yourself over how much the number on the scale has moved.

For that reason, make sure you fully think through the goals you set, as these guidelines can be applied to anything from weight loss, to scheduling meals or exercising more. Just remember, it's important to set goals you can act upon at least three times each week, ideally being able to do them everyday. This is especially important at the start of this process, as you will need to focus on getting into the mindset of developing a routine. While goals like 'walk to the shops instead of drive' will help your health, it's unlikely that you will be able to act upon them often enough to justify them being a focal point. So instead, save them for a later date to throw in as a secondary habit, or even better, try to consciously act upon them as and when they are appropriate.

Always remember: this is a new lifestyle, not an overnight fix, which is why the aim is slow cohesive progress, not radical drastic change. In the examples below, I have left out behaviours such as waking up earlier to have breakfast or similar changes in relation to how you eat, as although they are good goals to have, they may have already been introduced into your routine in relation to your diet, and at this point we are looking for additional improvements on your lifestyle on the whole.

Some examples of actions are:

- Add an extra portion of vegetables to every meal.
- Swap refined carbohydrates for wholegrain options for at least one meal a day.
- Drink more water by keeping a bottle on your desk, and aim to finish it by the end of the day.
- Find 15 minutes every night away from all distractions to relax or meditate.
- Replace your afternoon trip to the vending machine with a short walk instead.
- Go for a run or walk after work every night before dinner.
- Turn off all electronics an hour before bed so that you can unwind.
- If you are buying lunch, make sure you walk to get it instead of driving or getting it delivered.
- Have fruit in the afternoon instead of your usual high-sugar, processed snack.
- Spend 30 minutes everyday (or every other day) studying to further your career, learning a new language or taking up a hobby.
- Switch to using a smaller plate for meals to reduce portion sizes.

- Start everyday by drinking a glass of water, and have a glass 15 minutes before every meal to increase your water intake and decrease your volume of food consumed.

- Find ways to walk for at least 30 minutes each day, or set yourself a target amount of steps to reach.

That list should give you a few ideas, but your possibilities are pretty much endless depending on your personal situation. Now it is up to you to determine exactly what is important to you. I have kept the original three habits of eating more vegetables, drinking more water and walking more in there as well, as depending on how quickly you worked your way through this book, they may still be fairly new actions in your daily routine and therefore a good place to start.

Please note

One important consideration to make when setting goals is to ensure you focus on the behaviours you want, and not the ones you don't. In other words, base your goals on moving towards actions rather than away from them, and make sure they don't revolve around an "all or nothing" concept. Remember, this is all about positive change and not restriction, all while finding a balance between what you want and what your body needs. That's why you need to avoid unobtainable goals such as 'never eat chocolate again', as if you love chocolate, there's simply no way this goal will last.

Step 5:

Now that you have your strategies, it's time to determine which ones will form the foundation of your new habits, as these will become your main focus moving forward.

To do this I want you to work your way through the list you created in steps 3 and 4, then preferably in different colours, highlight the changes that are:

1)   Most important to you

2)   You think would have the biggest impact on improving on your health

Next, go through the list and honestly ask yourself on a scale of one to ten, how likely you are at this present point in time to be able to achieve this action and write the number next to it. Don't worry if you give certain actions a low score, even if they are an issue highlighted as most likely to have the biggest impact on your health. All it means is that your action either needs to be simplified, or you are not quite at a stage to pursue it yet. If this is the case don't be disheartened, just remember: 'a journey of a thousand miles begins with a single step', and having them on your list gives you something to work towards later when you are ready.

Once you have marked all your items, go back through the list. For goals scoring less than seven, see if you can think of a way to break them down further into steps that are more manageable. For instance, you could perceive eating a healthy diet based primarily around wholefoods as being the one change you would most like to achieve and would see the most benefit from. However, trying to change everything at once would be a daunting task, which is why in the previous section we broke the process up into four stages, focusing on one meal at a time before moving on to the next. The cumulative effect of these small steps added together will lead you to reach your overall goal in a manner that's not daunting or overwhelming, which is a perfect example of exactly why breaking down and simplifying processes is so important.

Another example is if you have never really been active before but want to start running three times a week. A good way to approach this would be to aim to run a short distance you know you are capable of completing. By doing so you remove the risk of doing too much on run one, allowing you to ease into it instead. Then, every week look to increase the distance a little bit further. Alternatively, you could start by walking the route three times a week, slowly building up to jogging, and then eventually running when you feel more comfortable.

Once you have done that, look over the new smaller goals and rescore them to see if they have improved, repeating this process until you are happy that larger actions can't be simplified any further.

Always remember: There's no denying that change is hard, which is why you need to do it gradually and prioritise what you choose to attempt first. That's why initially all that really matters is that you do something, as that will be what develops the habit. Because of that, the rate at which you progress is far less important than ensuring you stick to it.

Step 6:

With this in mind, I want you to choose one action to begin with, one change you know you can do without a doubt, and which will get you started on your journey to achieving your goal. To select this habit, go through your list of goals and choose the point you feel you can most easily achieve. Ideally, you would have marked it as either a nine or ten based on how confident you are that you can achieve it, coupled with being an action you can practice everyday. This is an essential part of the initial process, as in order to get into the routine of practicing habits it needs to be a regular occurrence, so leave pursuing less frequent habits to a later date.

Why are you doing it this way?

I know this may seem like a simplistic approach, but the purpose of choosing the easiest goal is to start you off with what I like to call 'quick wins'. These small, successful changes will be used to inspire and motivate you, putting you in a positive frame of mine by proving to yourself that you are capable of change. This quick win will give you a push to get started, overcoming the initial daunting hurdle of taking the first step. Although starting with one small habit may not seem like much, you will simultaneously be changing an aspect of your diet, giving you two things to focus on everyday, which combined, is more than enough to begin with.

Your chosen action could be something as small as adding a portion of vegetables to every meal, going for a 15-minute walk before dinner, or freeing up 30 minutes for yourself in the evening to read, study or simply relax. Another example is say you drink five cans of soda a day. To start with you could aim to reduce this to four, swapping one out for a glass of water. Then the next week reduce it to three and so on, and you could apply the same thinking to reducing the amount of sugar in your tea or coffee.

On their own, these changes may seem small and insignificant, but that's the entire point. They are simplified small actions that aren't overwhelming. Yet, they still develop healthy habits and over time, the cumulative impact they have will significantly add up, not just in the health benefits found through the new practice, but also in increasing your self-belief that change is possible.

Cues

When trying to develop new habits, a factor that will play a vital role in your success will be the implementation of a secondary action, or what's also known as a cue. These will act as both a reminder to perform your habit, all while simplifying the overall action, thereby reducing external factors that may tempt you into skipping it.

The cues you put in place will depend entirely on what you are attempting to do, so may take some thought on how you can streamline the process.

Some examples are:

- Packing a gym bag so you can go straight to the gym from work.

- Setting an alarm at certain times to remind you to perform the action e.g. to finish or fill up your water bottle.

- Placing reminders in your phone and scheduling the action as part of your day.

- Putting ingredients out on the table so you have them ready to make breakfast.
- Doing your shopping online so you have ingredients delivered to make meals and don't eat out.

To put this into perspective, let's revisit the example of putting all your ingredients for breakfast out the night before. To perform this cue you could put ready portioned oats in a bowl with some fruit on the counter. That way they are ready for you as soon as you get up, and act as a visual reminder you that you need to eat. In turn this will make it easier to get into the mindset of having breakfast every morning, thereby leading to the formation of new habit, that eventually becomes just another part of your everyday routine.

Another example could be adding an additional portion of vegetables to every meal. What you could do is chop and prepare the them when you get them home from the store, then keep them in a container in the fridge. That way they are ready for use, meaning the inconvenience of preparing them every time is removed, and you will have the added bonus of having a visual cue of seeing them in the container every time you open the fridge, acting as a reminder that you need to increase your intake.

Step 7:

Once you have chosen your habit for the next two weeks, I want you to practice it with the aim of consciously finding ways to achieve it every day. In order to be successful, it's essential you track and monitor your progress using a system of checks and balances, as this will be the only way to create a sense of accountability for your actions.

There are several ways to do this, with the quickest being to use the calendar on your phone, placing a green pin with the habit number on days you successfully achieve it, and a red pin on days you don't. Alternatively, you can use a notebook with a table and simply use a tick or cross system, but my personal preference is using a spreadsheet with a tally chart like the one below. The right way however is the one that works best for you.

Habit	Mon	Tues	Weds	Thurs	Fri	Sat	Sun
1							
2							
3							

You can get a copy of this 'Habit Tracker' tally chart in the downloadable activities pack at:

www.tailoredlifestyles.co.uk/activities

The 'reward' mechanism

I know that it is easy to think of something as simple as marking off an action on a calender as a stupid or redundant idea, but you will find that successfully marking off items in your grid everyday will actually give you a feel good moment every time you do. This acts as positive reinforcement, and associates actions taken with a reward (in this case the reward being that you feel good about yourself). This is an essential part of the formation of new habits, as that positive reinforcement gives you mental satisfaction, along with the motivation to continue in difficult times. You will also find that often simply the thought of having to mark an 'x' instead of a tick, or use a red dot instead of a green one, may be all it takes to go through with an action you were on the fence about skipping.

You can however put in place additional rewards to aid in accountability, which as with everything else, will vary from person to person, and be highly dependant on the goal or activity. For example; these could be anything from looking forward to a smoothie after working out, to the feeling gained from stepping on the scale each week and seeing you have lost weight, fitting into that old pair of jeans, buying something you want, an hour of guilt-free TV, or simply just the feel good moment of your success. The reward will come down to what you personally desire, and by ensuring it's something you really want, you can even focus on it during times of temptation, making it less likely you will give in.

To give you an example of this in action, sometimes after a long day the last thing I feel like doing is dragging myself to the gym and working out. Yet by simply thinking of how good I will feel afterwards, in most cases I'm able to get myself to go through with it. I have had to overcome this mindset many times, which is why I know full well that as soon as I start my workout, the feelings of not wanting to be there quickly pass. This in turn can help summon the internal motivation I need to push myself to go. To illustrate this point further, a study in 2002 at New Mexico State University looked at individuals who developed the habit of exercising. They found that while many started on a whim, the reason they continued was the craving of a specific reward they related to the action. The study found 92 percent of the participants in one group stuck to exercise as it made them 'feel good', whereas 67 percent in another group longed for that feeling of accomplishment gained from completing and progressing in their chosen activity.

Bear in mind though that since your aim should be to treat food as nourishment for your body, rather than because you deserve something, it's best not to use food as a reward. This is especially true if one of your main goals is weight loss, in which case it's best to look for non-food related rewards, that aren't counterproductive to your mental and physical progress.

It's important to take into consideration that while reward patterns can help develop new habits due to the positive emotions experienced, they can also be the cause of developing negative ones. That's why upon closer evaluation of your lifestyle, you may find many habits you believed to be rewarding are, in fact, hindering your progress. For example, going for a relaxing walk is far more rewarding in the long run than enabling emotional eating by having a sugary snack to treat yourself for your hard work at the office, and breaking these negative cycles of response and perceived reward will play a huge role in your success. Your bad habits only exist because at some point in time your brain perceived them as being a reward or something you wanted, meaning that by changing your reward mechanism you can replace bad habits with good ones.

"Habit is stronger than reason"

- George Santayana

Summarising the formation of new habits

In essence, forming new habits comes down to:
- Determining a goal or change you would like to make
- Putting together a cue to action it
- Practicing the action so it becomes routine
- Creating a reward you crave that motivates you to complete it

Studies however show that on their own, a cue and reward are often not enough to build a lasting habit, which is why it's important that the cue you choose not only triggers the action, but also creates a craving for the reward that follows. To be truly successful, your brain needs to start expecting and craving the reward, whether that's the feel good moment, a rush of energy and adrenaline, or the sense of accomplishment. When you reach this stage your actions will become automatic and driven by internal motivation.

Just to reiterate; you will only reach this point if you continually practice and follow through with your new habits, as repetition will be the only way to make new actions a part of your routine.

You can apply this basic formula to the formation of any new habit, but as an example, let's go with the idea that you want to start exercising more.

The cue would be taking your gym bag with you so that you can go straight from work, and the reward would be the post workout high of feeling good, a tasty smoothie, or whatever else appeals to you. Now by thinking about the reward, you start to anticipate it. Then in time, the anticipation creates a craving in your brain making it easier to motivate yourself to work out, as you look forward to the reward at the end.

It really is that simple and as you can see, there's no need to overcomplicate it or make it anymore difficult than it needs to be.

Anything else?

When practicing and developing new habits it's important to try to remove or minimise outside environmental factors that influence or spur on negative behaviours or impulses. On top of that, whenever you can, you need to consciously try and break cues that encourage negative behaviours. I know at first this may be difficult or inconvenient, but over time, it will get easier. For instance, if your goal is to avoid your afternoon trip to the bakery on your way home, then you could try and take another route. On the other side of this you could replace your afternoon cup of tea with a glass of water to remove the temptation of having those biscuits. Alternatively, if working out at home, make sure you start as soon as you get in. That way you avoid the risk of losing motivation by sitting down or getting distracted by the TV.

When deciding on what habits to pursue, try to think of all the potential barriers that come with it, the challenges that may arise, or anything that could potentially lead you off course. By anticipating the barrier, you can mentally prepare for the moment, and by doing so you will be more likely to respond accordingly.

Disclaimer

I'm not going to lie, not all new habits are fun to begin with and there will be times when you have to be very intentional about following through with them. But you just need to find a way to stick to them, no matter how challenging at times it may be. Even though it may not seem like it at first, over time, the new habits you are developing will become second nature. In the moments you struggle with motivation, refer back to your reasons for doing this and use those as your internal driving force to keep pushing yourself.

What now?

This marks the end of the activity based process where I wanted you to read it step by step, so from here feel free to continue reading as you normally would. Over the course of this programme it will be essential you regularly refer back to these pages, just to ensure you know exactly how you should be approaching your journey.

"Being challenged in life is inevitable, being defeated is optional."

- Roger Crawford

Other useful tools and strategies

Monitoring Progress

At the end of each week, it's useful to spend some time reflecting and evaluating what happened. Look at areas in which you were both successful and unsuccessful, in order to uncover any patterns or trends. Is there a recurring cue you never considered that's leading you off track? What did you do well? Where could you have done better? What difficult situations did you face and how could you deal with them better next time? What have you learned about yourself that you didn't know you were capable of doing? And what are you going to focus on doing differently next week?

Forming new habits takes time, which is why engaging in personal reflection is such a vital part of the process. Not only will it help you to develop and grow, but in addition it will allow you to use yourself as a support system for positive reinforcement, reminding you that you can and will do it, as well as regularly remembering your reasons for starting in the first place.

Alternatively, you may want to discuss your progress with a friend, family member or even an online community/support network. Talk about how you did, what you found hard, how you could do better and what steps you will take next. As I keep stressing, everyone is different, so you need to find what works best for you and which outlet creates the most positive accountability to help you stick to your goals. Sometimes just knowing you need to check in or tell someone you achieved your goal for the day can be the boost you need to follow through with it, and maybe those you confide in are even on a similar journey and you can help each other. Just letting them know why you couldn't do it may be the reassurance you need to remember tomorrow is another day, where you can and will get back on track.

Wins and losses journal

Another form of accountability I like to incorporate is what I call a "wins and losses" journal. The purpose of this is to make a note of every time you either gave in or overcame temptation. Time and date it along with a quick description of what happened and how you responded. Keep these notes in a notebook, on your phone, or in any form that is easiest for you to review at the end of each week during your reflection. You may even want to keep them in a separate tab on the spreadsheet you are using to track how you are doing in other areas, as that way you keep everything in once place and make it easy to refer back to.

One of the main benefits of this journal is that it keeps a record of what happened, which gives you more insight when looking for patterns or trends in the decisions you have made. The journal keeps you from having to rely on your memory, which is especially useful when comparing a few weeks at a time to see how you are progressing. You are likely to find correlations between circumstances and outside factors you never even considered, and be able to use your findings to help remove or avoid those negative influences in the future. Looking back at it can also give you a sense of achievement, as you can see all the times you overcame adversity and challenges. In addition you may benefit from keeping a note in your journal about times you feel the urge to resume old habits. Simply by taking a moment to write it down before acting upon it will highlight that it still exists in your mind. This could be the internal motivation standing between whether you stay strong, give in, or relapse. This can relate to anything from quitting smoking, to drinking or eating processed foods, as writing it down forces you to take a moment and think twice about what you truly want. At the end of the day, your journey is just as important as the destination, which is why personal growth is a big part of developing a healthy lifestyle. By regularly checking in with yourself, you will not only learn more about who you are, but also what you are capable of.

Pros and cons list

If you are still struggling with motivation or sitting on the fence about whether or not to go through with something, then try creating a pros and cons list.

Depending on where you are mentally, this could be useful in times of doubt for starting and continuing the process, or even when working on a particular habit. You can even use this strategy in other aspects of your life.

To use this list write down what you are contemplating at the top of a piece of paper. Below that write all the positives you could gain from pursuing it on one side, and all the negatives on the other. This might include anything from better health, to more energy, saving money, reducing risk of diseases, losing weight etc., whereas the other side may be all about things you perceive as losing or giving up. Such as watching less TV, getting up earlier, spending time cooking, exercising, or being more organised with planning and scheduling. Hopefully from doing this exercise you will be able to see that what you have to gain far outweighs the small changes you initially view as sacrifices. This method may help you not only get started, but keep you going in times of doubt as well.

You can access a ready-made list in the downloadable activities pack at **www.tailoredlifestyles.co.uk/activities.**

"Be not afraid of going slowly, be afraid only of standing still."

- Chinese proverb

Moving forward

Step 8:

After two weeks of practicing your habit, it's now time to progress further in your journey and add a second goal. To do so, go back to your list and select the habit you feel will most likely lead to the next 'quick win'. By doing this again, you will continue to build your confidence. Ideas you originally ranked as seven or lower will eventually seem less intimidating and more achievable, meaning that in time, you can start progressing towards them. For the next two weeks, follow the same procedures, keeping track of whether or not you achieved your habits, and keeping your wins and losses journal up to date. Then at the end of each week re-evaluate to see how you found practicing more than one habit at a time. From here on out your aim should be to add a new habit every two weeks, however, make sure that when adding new habits that you continue to practice your previous ones until they are no longer something you need to force or think about.

If at any point you feel overwhelmed or like you need longer to focus on what you are doing, then don't pressure yourself into progressing further. What's important is moving at a rate that is manageable, instead of overwhelming. Ultimately progress is still progress, regardless of how small it may be. But with that being said, it's essential you keep pushing yourself, as fundamentally, that's the only way you grow. So don't let the fact that you know you can dial it back to act as an incentive to ignore your exercise or drift off course, as it is an easy excuse to use, that in many ways can hold you back.

With all things considered this process will be all about finding the right balance, which is why it's essential that you don't let one bad day push you into a state of mind where you feel like its all too much or think you can't do it. When bad days happen, simply write them off, get a good night's sleep, and reassess in the morning.

Reassessing goals

At the end of every two-week period go back to your original list and re-evaluate the scores you gave each goal. You will find that as you progress, your perception of what you feel capable of achieving will improve, and the prospect surrounding the lower-scored challenges will become far less daunting. You may also have thought of new goals you would like to achieve, so use this time to add them to the list.

Step 9:

At the end of the first four weeks you should be comfortable practicing multiple habits. Your confidence in your abilities should be higher, you will be used to creating and managing accountability, along with tracking, monitoring and evaluating your progress. By now it's likely you will have dealt with several setbacks, and hopefully from that you developed a new outlook of resilience, and got yourself back on track. That's why now is the time to challenge yourself further, as you really start progressing within your goal.

The purpose of the 'quick wins' was to boost your confidence and prove to yourself that you are capable of change, so now you can shift your focus to a potentially larger challenge. From your list of goals marked at least a seven or eight out of ten, pick the one you feel is likely to have the biggest positive impact on your overall health. This challenge will definitely be harder than the previous ones and push you further out of your comfort zone, with potentially more setbacks. But through the process of slowly building up to it, you will be far more prepared and ready to handle it, even if it takes more effort. You just need to believe you can do it.

If however you feel like you are not quite ready for the next big step, then don't feel disheartened. There's nothing wrong with sticking to the habits you are currently practicing for a couple more weeks, or adding another 'quick win' so you can continue taking smaller steps. If you don't feel quite ready for a bigger challenge yet, but still want to push yourself further, then you may even want to try incorporating two new smaller goals at once, or even another 'quick win' combined with some additional secondary targets.

Leading up to this point has been all about making you accountable for your own actions, which is why I'm leaving the judgment on which direction to take up to you. Above all, this is your journey, and because of that only you can decide what you truly want and is right for you.

With that being said though, rushing this process or trying to do too much too soon is a recipe for disaster, which is why

I can't stress enough that you should only add new habits and actions when you feel comfortable enough to progress. Ignoring this advice will likely lead to relapses and feelings of overwhelm, which are exactly the feelings you are trying to avoid.

Remember that forming new habits takes time, and unfortunately doing so often takes far longer than you would like it to, or feel that it should. The reality is they simply can't be forced, with studies showing that depending on how big of a change they are, new habits can take anything from 21 to 66 days to be formed. That's why patience is a vital skill you need to develop throughout this process, but trust me, with continued perseverance, your new actions will eventually become automatic and integrated within you. What may be challenging at first, will eventually just become an everyday automatic reaction, and part of a routine you do without thinking.

This is why you need to continue practicing your habits on a daily basis, and they should only be removed from your progress charts as and when you are confident that acting on them no longer requires any conscious thought. There may even be times when you relapse or fall back into other bad habits, in which case you will need to refocus your attention on getting them right.

Recap

The steps are as follows:

- List why this is important to you along with what you would like to achieve.

- Draw up a list of actions and using a one to ten method, score them on how confident you are that you can achieve them.

- Following that, choose one habit to start with, selecting the easiest as you aim for your first 'quick win'.

- Keep a record as a form of accountability and reference guide for whether or not you successfully practiced your new habits.

- Keep a wins and losses journal to add another layer of evaluation and accountability.

- Every two weeks look at adding a new habit.

- Keep practicing your habits until you no longer have to consciously think about doing them (could take between 21 to 66 days).

- If you struggle with a habit, strip it back, modify or simplify it.

Eventually you will reach a point in your journey where you habitually start making decisions that are the most beneficial for your health and therefore you no longer need to actively focus on developing them as habits. But until then, continue repeating this process until you achieve the health you desire. Your journey doesn't stop there though, and you can continue to progress in all areas of life, with a new found vigour and health.

"Every successful individual knows that his or her achievement depends on a community of persons working together"

- Paul Ryan

Community

Having a support network there for you every step of your journey can play a huge role in your success, and because of that, I decided to set up a 'Become a better you' online community for all those embarking on this process. The idea of creating a platform where people could engage with others who are on the same path is a concept that really appealed to me, and personally I think it's an exciting addition to this programme, especially knowing that there will be people from around the world you can engage with on a daily basis, who are on a similar path and in the same stages of their journey as you.

My idea behind this community was to create a judgement-free zone, where anyone is welcome to share their thoughts, opinions, triumphs and setbacks, or even discussions on recipes, TV shows, or anything else of interest. Where they can use the platform to check in, share whether they successfully completed their habits for the day and hold not only themselves, but also others accountable for their actions.

You are not only welcome to join and take part, but to make the most of this book I highly recommend that you do. It will be a great way to see that you are not alone, and there are others out there just like you.

I really want this community to thrive, but just like anything else, it will only be as successful as the members who take part, so you really will only get out what you put in.

This community is free to access and will remain that way, so use it to share stories, meet friends, track your journey and help others.

You can join in at www.tailoredlifestyles.co.uk/forums

Closing thoughts

Well there you have it; we have reached the end of this process.

I'd like to take a moment to thank you for reading this book, and I hope you enjoyed it as much as I enjoyed writing it.

I'm confident that by following the steps and information within, that you will not only look, but also feel better than you ever have before, as you take back your health and become the best version of yourself.

If you have any questions about health, nutrition, dieting, fitness, or anything featured, you can get in touch with me at any time at:

byron@tailoredlifestyles.co.uk.

Offering this service is my way of giving back to those struggling with the same journey I was on a few years ago, and I dedicate some time each day to answer questions from anyone who needs my support.

Alternatively, if you would like additional support, I offer one-to-one Lifestyle and Weight Loss Coaching, as well as my '8 weeks to a better you' Healthier Wellbeing Programme, which I developed around the information in this book.

The programme itself takes all the key principles and delivers them through a series of weekly online seminars with tailored guidance, accountability and support every step of the way. All while be based around a supportive community of others who are on the same journey.

Like I said at the start, I designed this book and process around the help and guidance I wish was available to me when I started my journey, which is why I set up this course to offer exactly that.

Eiither way, remember to book your free 'start your weight loss journey' break through session with me over Skype, where I will help you map out the exact steps you need to get started.

You can find out more about booking your session or my coaching at: www.tailoredlifestyles.co.uk

Once again, thank you, and I wish you all the best in your journey.

Byron Morrison

$7 \times 1.54 = 10.78$